# CRITICAL THINKING

## EFFECTIVE
## MENTAL HEALTH TRAINING
## TO ENHANCE PERFORMANCE

Trawn Barrington

ISBN: 979-8-89075-009-9

# DESCRIPTION

A 3-part story based on true events. The novel works on dealing with challenges in your daily life, small or big, and useful ways of overcoming those circumstances in a beneficial way. With easy-to-understand material that caters to all ages and genders, this is a book that is relatable and has lessons on dealing with mental health worldwide.

Useful in business, exercise science, and social science classrooms as well as other similar majors and courses from high school to graduate programs at a college or a university. A great read for all athletes enhancing team-building skills. The novel has been developed with a 16-week activity plan to engage students in the classroom. The book can be a good part of an academic curriculum or lesson plan because it lets students think and be more focused on the details of a task at hand, which is necessary for every major or area of academic study. Includes readers notepad with every purchase.

# MENTAL HEALTH TRAINING TIPS

## (Recommended For Everyday Use)

Many of us let our environment and people's expectations determine our future outcomes. No one cares. Keep going. You were not born to be average, so why settle? If you want to reach your maximum potential, do not allow someone to tell you that you cannot do something. The strongest have the hardest battles; however, they overcome them. Make a choice to keep moving forward and let success be your greatest achievement.

# 10 DAILY SELF-TALK SLOGANS TO FOLLOW

1. No matter what situation you are in, confidence moves mountains.
2. A small circle is always better than a big circle.
3. Train your mind to not overthink by using meditation and positive thoughts.
4. There is never a wrong time to do the right thing.
5. Success is not based on money; it is based on stability.
6. To overcome daily obstacles, always remember that achievements are based off of 99% effort and 1 % skill.
7. Challenges are overwhelming to those who are weak.
8. A man or woman can only be at their best when they can block out liabilities.
9. The richest people in the world started with an idea. What is yours?
10. If you have done the work and life is not going as planned, focus on small changes.

# PART 1

–

# BASED ON A TRUE STORY

As the buses passed and the casino lights flashed, it was time for the day to start. In a small-town part of the mega city of Toronto, there was Rexdale. With a population of just about 120,00 people, ¼ of every person was living below the poverty line. The town had been famous for west Indian food spots and the horse racing over at the Woodbine Race Track, located beside 3 colorful tall buildings. The buildings included a blue building, a yellow building, and a red building. The 3 buildings were better known to be on the street of Queens Plate. These buildings were so tall and colorful that you could see them while on highway 27 or coming from Mississauga, passing the famous Mr. Jerk Jamaican cuisine. A diverse community surrounded by skyscrapers, the people were predominantly Asian and African Canadians. Throughout the 3 buildings, there were refugees and immigrants who would live in the low-income apartments. These minorities were hard-working men and women whom every day tried to do the best for their families. The only problem with good, hard-working people who lived in low-income areas was that they were faced with adversity every day. Adversity to feed their families, get government assistance, and be educated to be able to move out of the projects.

In the yellow building right in the middle of the blue and red on the 3rd floor in apartment 315 lived a newly born baby named Andrew and a single mom named Kesha. Andrew's Dad, Ben, and his mom, Kesha, broke up right after he was born. I guess there was no surprise because 1 month after Andrew was born, Ben had another baby with his mistress. Ben was now on his 3rd child in 3 years with 3 different women. Andrew was too young to know what was going on; he only knew it was going to be him and his mom in that little apartment in the yellow building.

As Andrew grew a little older and started to go to kindergarten, he was able to form friendships on the playground. Andrew began to talk to a boy named Seth, who was a couple of years older than him and was in his aftercare program until his mom picked him up after work. Seth had a younger brother and a younger sister who sometimes attended the aftercare program that accommodated children from JK to 5th grade. Seth was energetic, but he tended to hang out with the wrong crowd.

The aftercare facility was located at the main entrance of two elementary schools, Humberwood Downs, which was a public school that had a diverse population. The second school was Holy Child, which had mostly Latin and African Canadians. Both schools comprised about 1500 students from the 1st grade to the 8th grade. The school was located a 5-minute drive from the colored buildings. The school was beside a park, a small river under a bridge, townhouses, and a big bus station for the city. As time flew by, Andrew was around the age of six in the 1st grade. 1st grade was not a big adjustment because Andrew was still a part of the aftercare program, which was located at the public school near his home address.

In the years after his father left, Andrew was still trying to figure out who to look up to, how to dress, and how to make friends. He wished his Dad was there to help him throughout his early school years. One day on a sunny weekday, there were children running around, birds chirping, and a graceful breeze on a peaceful day. Andrew was playing a Yugioh card game with the deck his mom got him for Christmas. He and his friends were going at it, having fun and having a great time.

It was getting competitive. As time passed, there were some bullies who came up to Andrew and his friends and took his Yugioh deck from him. They ran so fast, and they had to be at least in the 3rd or 4th grade, a few years older than Andrew. Andrew was surprised that one of his friends, Seth, witnessed what happened by luck. Seth was an older kid around ages 8 or 9 years old. He saw his friend needed help and ran to get those cards back. Seth had more respect in the school since he had a lot of friends and he was popular.

As the weeks passed, Andrew would commute to school with his mom in the morning and leave in the afternoon, regularly attending the after-school program with his favorite teacher Cara. Cara was wonderful and was always engaged with the children, a great woman overall. Andrew was picked up later that evening from Cara. 5 minutes from the colored apartments, Kesha got her son from daycare in an old Chevrolet 5-seater. Kesha and Andrew were discussing what should be eaten that night.

As they settled in, there were 3 other friends in apartment 315. Roach 1, 2, and 3. Used to roaches, Andrew killed them, and Kesha called the exterminator for the next day. Andrew avoided going outside at his apartment unless the ice cream truck was coming or it was a nice day to get fresh air. Within his apartment, a typical day would be dogs barking, crackheads coming to re-up, and thugs selling drugs. Andrew came down the elevator and went outside on his bike. He was approached quickly by his other friend in daycare. Mark was around the same age and lived on the 1st floor of the 15-story building. There was a commotion outside, and there were a lot of neighbors whispering. Andrew was shy and was only at the age of 7 now, so he would not dare to speak up in grown business. Mark's mom was well known, and she was close to a lot of people, especially Seth's mom. As the commotion spread and got louder, Andrew's ears got bigger. Mark's volume got louder. Mark told Andrew, "Seth is no longer with us." Andrew had nothing to say. Trying to process death as a 7-year-old is not as easy as a developed adult. Andrew asked Mark, "Are you sure?" Mark cried, "Yes. I'm sure!"

Earlier, it was discussed about the school Andrew attended, which was both public and catholic, located near a bridge and a river, about a 3-minute walk from the school and right where Seth helped Andrew get his Yugioh cards. Seth was found dead by homicide, and his body was floating through the river under the bridge. As the days passed, Seth's younger sister and brother had not returned to school. Another year older, Andrew was now in the 3rd grade. He was still a part of the aftercare program and now began a basketball program every Thursday night for an hour. Andrew was able to be a part of something and build his confidence. Kesha dropped Andrew off at school on a calm day while she rushed to work. She made sure he was well acquainted with his surroundings and got to his class.

After the day was over, Andrew walked through a steep hill with a high ceiling, near the gymnasium, beside a small library on his way to daycare. Andrew saw one of the people in daycare who he was familiar with getting beat up by some older children in the 5th grade. They kicked him and punched him several times while he tried to defend himself. Bystanders passed by; people watched but did not intervene. It was not until the principal came that there was a stop to the beatdown of this undeserving light skin boy. Andrew returned the next day to learn those kids were suspended; he later got into an argument with his daycare teacher, cussing her out. The Thursday of his basketball session, he got in trouble for bullying a kid at the program. Andrew felt as if the boy had female parts and would make fun of his appearance. Andrew got scolded outside of the facility near the parking lot by his mom, and he got upset and kicked in his mom's car, denting the front bumper. Andrew was a good kid, but now his environment was rubbing off on him negatively.

A couple of weeks passed, and he came to school. In the morning, there were children fighting at recess; he continued to walk around the corner of the school, not sure where to fit in. He saw there was another fight going on with a bat, leaving one student in the hospital with life-threatening injuries. Andrew left school, and as he was on his 5-minute trip home with his mom after she picked him up, there was a group of 7 or 8 6th grade children from the catholic school beating up a young black man at the park.

Andrew started seeing his father more, from never seeing him to seeing him twice a month. Ben now had 4 children within 6 years with 4 different women, and he tried to reunite with them. Every few weeks, Andrew would go to a tall apartment building similar to the yellow building he lived in and would stay there Saturday and Sunday in the city of St. Catherine's, a commute about an hour from Toronto. Andrew was there with his stepbrother Peter, his little brother Pat, and his sister Amy. There were awkward exchanges at times and not a real bond since Andrew was forced into the situation by his Dad's actions. Ben would pick the children up or make sure they all got a way to come to his home by train. You would think Ben was a great father figure. When the children got home at the apartment in St. Catherine's, Ben would be absent

– probably having sex with his wife, possibly watching a movie, or maybe even doing business.

The only thing that Andrew knew was he probably would see his father in three situations. When it was time to come to his house, when it was time to eat a frozen meal, and when it was time for everyone except the youngest Amy to go back to their mom's house. Andrew had no father figure when he was born to when he was a young child visiting on the weekends to see his father.

On one of the weekends, it was raining and was rather cloudy. Ben did his usual routine, picking up his children like a great father would. Ben brought his kids back to the house and disappeared until it was time to eat a frozen meal. He did not cook and always would raise his voice to assert his authority. Love was a word that did not exist ever in that home. In one of the rooms, there was a bunk bed that could fit 2 people. Andrew, Peter, and Pat were in the room just talking about nothing like regular kids do. Amy was asleep when Ben and his wife were nowhere to be found for hours at a time. Peter was 12, Andrew was 9, Pat was 9, and Amy was 6 at the time. As Andrew was sitting next to his brother, Pat, who was in the middle of the lower bunk bed next to Peter, Peter gave Andrew and Pat instructions.

The instructions were to perform a sexual act on Pat and then on Peter, then Pat would reciprocate the act. Misguided and still with no guidance or father figure, the act was performed. With no guidance and no understanding of how disgusting and abusive this behavior was, it was swept under the rug. No questions asked, and it was never discussed after that day. Andrew was 10 years old and had already been through the worst of the worst, from crime, poverty, substance abuse, and molestation co-existing around him. As another year went by, Andrew began to get angrier. Talking back to his mom and disrespecting her. Andrew was no longer a passive, quiet kid. With no father around, Kesha called Tyson.

Tyson was a big 6'2 bearded business owner who also was Andrew's godfather. When Tyson was called, nothing good came out of it. 9/10 times it meant someone was about to get a whooping. In this instance, it was Andrew. Every time Andrew's mom tried to hit him, it did not work because he would rebel. She would call his godfather Tyson. Tyson was not one to play; he would beat Tyson with a belt and a hanger until there were scars left.

Andrew never spoke about how his father treated him after they got to his Dad's house – what he witnessed or the abuse he encountered. He stayed mute for a lot of years, trying to force himself to forget the bad memories. He became angry inside, infuriated with his circumstances, and wanted to make a better life for himself. If his mom knew that maybe Kesha would not allow Tyson to whip her son, maybe she would do a little more to figure out why there was so much anger and aggression. When Andrew was at school, he was in aftercare, minding his business, listening to music on a cd player with his friends. Everyone was dancing and having a good time.

There was one kid named Anthony. He was in the 4th grade, the same age as Andrew, always loud, and always acted like he was someone better than his peers. He decided one day to throw the hot rice pudding that he was eating at Andrew. Andrew, already built up with aggression and anger from his circumstances, said, "Today is the day." He followed Anthony because he ran away, knowing he was wrong. Near the library where James the light skin boy got beat up a few years back.

Andrew punched him all over from head to toe. Threw him to the ground and started to kick him.After that day, Andrew had begun to go on a negative path that would lead him to prison or death. Between the years of the 2nd grade to the 5th grade, Andrew had been well known by all the principals at the school; even the secretary had known Andrew by his first name, which was not good. Andrew had racked up over 10 suspensions in 3 years. At the age of 12, the teachers had constantly been seen talking about Andrew not wanting him in their classes. Andrew's suspensions would be for disruption, fighting, and misconduct in a school. Andrew had thrown objects at students. Andrew had been seeking attention. Maybe it was from his father, maybe it was from his mother, letting her know these circumstances were too much. Andrew had just wanted to be a child and have fun; however, his childhood was passing him by.

Andrew would go back to his apartment, and there was a young boy named James. He played outside a lot and was around the usual drug dealers and crack heads who loitered the area. A few weeks later, James was pronounced dead after an incident with the cops. This had shaken the apartment complex because his mom had been so caring and had tried her best to get her son on the right path. It had been a relaxed day that evening after hearing the news. The usual, children shooting each other with bb guns and firecrackers, kids getting beat up at the community park, and the smell of poverty had loomed in the air.

Later that year, Andrew had discovered something. His teacher Mr. Taylor had been fundraising which he does every year. The profits had come from books, magazines, and stickers, which could be purchased by the family and friends of each student. All the profits had gone to a charity for children. Mr. Taylor had accumulated about 200$ so far and kept his earnings in the cabinet at the end of the classroom on the 3rd floor at Andrew's public school. Andrew, every single day, would see Mr. Taylor adding money and, at times, forgetting to lock it. When the classes were dismissed, Andrew would take a couple dollars out of the fundraising jar each week. He had eventually accumulated nearly 100$, almost half of his earnings. Naive about the situation and on the verge of getting suspended from the public school, Andrew had not thought he would get caught.

One day as Andrew made his way upstairs to the 3rd floor, passing the big windows on the staircase, he had stumbled past a kid who had gotten initiated into a gang by 5 or 6 people, and Andrew had finally come to the 3rd floor. It was a story that everyone had been listening to. Andrew had struggled to stay engaged and had been nervous because Mr. Taylor said he was missing some money. The money had been gone and nowhere to be found. While Mr. Taylor was talking to the class, he had been directly looking into the eyes of Andrew. Mr. Taylor had been a smart man and could see that Andrew had been nervous. After class, he had told Andrew he could tell by his reaction that he stole the money. Mr. Taylor had given Andrew two options: he pays back the 100$, or he calls the police. Andrew had been relieved he could pay it back without getting in trouble with his mom or the police. Andrew had paid 12$ every week for about 9 weeks. 12$ was his allowance, so that's all Andrew had had to pay every week to Mr. Taylor.

Andrew had still been having trouble at home, and Kesha said it was time to make a change. She said, "I cannot afford it, but whatever I have, I will use it for my son in private school for the next few years." Andrew came home to a home-cooked meal. Kesha was a strong woman and a hard worker. She was an immigrant from London, England, and she had been to several countries. Guyana was where Kesha's family ties were from. That home-cooked meal Andrew got was really good. Curry chicken and roti were one of his favorites. You could tell Andrew was an island boy at heart even though he was born in Toronto.

Toronto is such a beautiful city. If you ever get a chance to go there, you should. Toronto is a diverse city. Some of the greatest entertainers come there, a great sports atmosphere and the views from the high-rise buildings looking down on the city are mesmerizing. Just a reminder, the legal age is 19. If you like to dance and see attractive people, you can attend the Caribbean festival in August near the beautiful beach near downtown Toronto. Anyway, back to the story.

Andrew was born in Toronto, and he would come to the Caribana festival with his Dad's side of the family for a couple of summers on the weekend. After going to Caribana, he might go back to his Dad's house with some of his siblings. At his Dad's house, now upgraded from the apartment in St. Catherine's, he would come in and see the beautiful interior, but there was no home feeling. Andrew wanted something better than the poor yellow building he lived in with constant violence.

As he continued to inspect the home, his Dad let him get settled. Andrew and his brothers were in the room playing with the old Nintendo 64 Mario carts. Andrew, Pat, and Peter paused for a second. They heard a commotion going on. Ben said to his wife Kate why are you always arguing in front of these kids. Kate resulted in assaulting Ben and throwing a knife at him. The kids went back to playing their game. Over the next few months, the kids came over a few times each month and were put to work. They were doing construction and lifting up stones with their Dad. As they finished up working on a shed and renovating a house, weeks later, they learned the house was being sold. Andrew's best memory of that house was that when he came over, he was never told he was loved. When his mom got him a bag, his Dad picked it up and threw it on the ground, and all his sunscreen squirted in the bag. Coming to that house, Andrew saw his Dad in the room for hours when he was the only one at the house. Staying in the basement alone, far away from home, made Andrew sad inside. On to the next home. Now, this home was magnificent and had a lot of beauty to the structure.

Ben was a big-time engineer and had acquired assets. "Look at this beautiful house with a 2-door garage with a beautiful 2-million-dollar house next door!" His wife loved to brag about it. Her property's value was increasing. There had to be great energy in that house for Andrew and his siblings. Let's talk about these memories. They had to be better than the old house. Well, this is what happened. Ben was a dictator. When he called you by your name, he did not want to repeat himself. Andrew and Amy were bonding until he started shouting Amy's name. He had verbally abused her and made her cry more times than Andrew could count. Andrew and Pat would lay back on the couch in the basement to watch a movie. Boom! Boom! Boom! You could hear loud footsteps. Ben was coming down the stairs. He began shouting at Andrew and Pat. He said, "This is not your house. Get up! Do not get comfortable here! Lay back at your mom's house."

Pat told Andrew, "I thought this was our house," as he chuckled. Andrew began to chuckle after. Laughter was something that was constantly done to overcome anger; however, sometimes, it was okay to get angry. This was one of many examples of Ben not showing love and care for his kids. If you had ever studied psychology or similar subjects you may have come across Maslow's hierarchy of needs which discusses a theory of human motivation in which every human being seeks self-actualization, esteem, love and belonging, safety needs, and psychological needs. When there is a gap in those human needs, a person can be constantly seeking that fulfillment.

As Andrew transitioned into the 6th grade, he began to enter a private school. This was a way for his mom to help him overcome his issues at the public school. The private school lasted 2 years, and throughout those years, he engaged in a lot of prayers, 1 on 1 learning, and public speaking. Throughout these two years, Andrew enrolled in a group session for troubled youth every Wednesday night at 6 PM. The discussion would be on ways for kids to channel emotions, whether it was happiness, grief, or anger. This program was a good stepping stool for Andrew to get on the right track. His mom's sacrifice might have paid off. He was able to not get suspended anymore and show growth. There was a Sargent-type principal who was a man of God. Mr. Hughes, he would even beat the kids if they got out of line. Kesha deserved an award for how she was still struggling to pay rent in roach-infested, poor immigration housing and still sent her son to private school. There was one thing that needed to be changed: the environment.

Andrew was now 14, and his mom knew it was time for a change. The lease was over. Where could the next move be? Kesha's new lease was not in the area. 2 years after enrolling in private school, the high school that Andrew would be required to attend was a school known for lockdowns, shootings, and stabbings. Kesha's move was in impeccable timing. She moved to a city called Brampton, a 30-minute drive from Toronto.

Andrew was in the 8th grade now. Andrew was in a new environment surrounded by a lot of Asian Americans. He met 2 guys named Alonzo and Tyler. They both played Jr. Varsity football for the city. This school was a great place. There were no fights. Everyone was a part of a club or sports team in middle school. Andrew joined the basketball, wrestling, volleyball, and flag football team. You could say Andrew was engaged in sports. He put all of his adversity behind him and continued to participate in sports right before he entered high school. Andrew was spoken to by Alonzo and Tyler about joining the Jr. Varsity football team as there were winter tryouts coming up. The only experience playing sports for Andrew was Thursday nights back in Toronto and his fall season playing sports at his new public school. He said, "Sure, why not? I do not mind trying something new."

He knew he had overcome struggles that made him feel fearless. Andrew entered an indoor practice facility and began to work with some of the players on agility and coordination. His conditioning was improving every Saturday that his mom took him. Being at a school that was in Brampton allowed for a peaceful experience compared to the last 15 years. Andrew would stay at his aunt Shelly's house after school until his mom was able to pick him up. Aunt Shelly's house was fun. He would have a home-cooked meal from his grandma and watch movies with his uncle. Aunt Shelly had a nice 3-story house with 3 bedrooms and a backyard, something Andrew was not used to seeing before. Kesha would make her way from work in Toronto to Brampton to get her son as soon as she could. Andrew became a big-time name in his new public school. Andrew would do a lot of reading and learn how to interact with his peers more without feeling hostility. It was overall a more positive experience for Andrew and his family. Andrew was able to win a middle school flag football championship and became a starter on the volleyball, basketball, and wrestling team.

In the 8th grade, there was a showcase in front of the students for the wrestling team. They did not allow Andrew to wrestle because he was the best at the school, and he was destroying the other middle schoolers in practice. Andrew met a couple of people he was close with and was able to grow some friendships with them. Andrew was still on edge everywhere he walked. He felt like he was waiting for something to happen. He was waiting for a fight to break out or for someone he knew to die by homicide. At the time, he still had PTSD from living in the project housing in Toronto. Andrew would have a spot where he would go at lunch if it was not a pizza day or if he did not have a packed lunch. There was a plaza about a 5-minute walk from where his public school was. They had the best fries and sandwiches nearby.

This public school felt like heaven to Andrew. There were dance parties. The school was overall more engaging. After Alonzo and Tyler told Andrew to try out for Jr. Varsity, Andrew made the team and worked his way up the ranks to become a starter for the city of Brampton. The football culture in Brampton was big. Brampton had a large history of winning many championships in football and wanted to continue that culture. Andrew and his teammates traveled on a coach bus and built unity. Andrew felt like he was a part of something productive and felt great for the first time. That year Andrew made the playoffs with his team but failed to win a championship. Regardless, he overcame adversity and was on his path to going to high school in less than 6 months.

A few years before Andrew attended private school, he was not sure he would make it to high school. Andrew thought he might end up like Seth or some of the other misguided children in Toronto. Overcoming adversity was like a logo for Andrew as he was becoming more resilient. Andrew had not seen or heard from his father in months. Ben would tell Andrew, "He is coming to Brampton to see his friend Paul so he guesses he could make an appearance to see his son play football. You can say Ben was an inconsiderate man who prioritized his wife and friends over his kids. Later that year, after the sports in school and Jr. Varsity football was over, Andrew was able to get an opportunity to travel to Texas to compete for the under 16 national football team vs. team USA. This was a big opportunity for Andrew and Kesha. Kesha saved up almost 500$ to get Andrew to enjoy this opportunity.

The trip was for a week in the summer, which his team drove across the border until they got to Texas. Texas was a new experience for a 15-year-old who only traveled to Guyana when his grandfather died in a hit-and-run homicide and Jamaica in the 1st grade briefly with his aunt. Texas was a football fanatic state. Country to the core and high in their values and community unity. When the bus arrived with 40 of his teammates, Andrew was embraced by some big country town representatives. The Americans let the team settle in their rooms and treated everyone, including team USA to a fattening, greasy Texas cookout. An unhealthy cookout may not be the best idea especially before early morning practice; some of the players felt sluggish after dinner. The next 6 days included practice, events, a tour of the city, and the conclusion of a big showdown game in a nice stadium. Team Canada vs. Team USA for all the chips and bragging rights. The game was extremely close; however, team USA came out victorious. It was a long drive back, but the experience made it worth it and built confidence amongst the team.

Andrew was back in Brampton, considering what high school to attend in the next 3 months. The closest to Brampton Tower Apartments was a school called Brampton Centennial Secondary school. There was only one issue for Andrew. There was no football team; the only contact sport was rugby.

"What to do now?" That thought ran through Andrew's mind and kept running through his mind as he tried to set up his high school experience. Some of his classmates from the 8th grade were discussing a new school in the making, which had a turf football field and was about to have all brand-new labs and facilities. This school was called David Suzuki Secondary school. Andrew and Kesha spoke about possible options on a Monday afternoon in their apartment in Brampton after school. This apartment was on the 9th floor, surrounded by 5 or 6 other skyscrapers, nearby a 100-store mall, and near the bus station. There was not much crime in the area where Kesha and Andrew relocated.

There was one homicide, security had gotten beat up, and some drugs were sold, but it was like night and day compared to the yellow building. Andrew told his mom he did not want to attend the nearby high school and would like to attend the big, fancy school that was almost done being constructed. Andrew knew if he wanted to go far in football, he should not restrict himself to the school zone. Andrew told his mom that his middle school coach would assist in developing the new football program, which would be a blessing for his development. Andrew and Kesha decided to use their aunt's address, who lived near the new school, and it was confirmed that Andrew would be a grizzly in the fall.

As the summer passed, there was a new development in the school's infrastructure. David Suzuki himself had attended the grand opening of the school he was named after. The ribbon was cut, the faculty was staffed, and the students were assigned to their classrooms for the year. Coach Patterson, a former CFL player and the head coach for the championship flag football team Andrew attended in the 8th grade, was the new offensive coordinator at David Suzuki Secondary school. The turf field was still in the initial stages. Construction was still being done daily to make sure it met city inspection. A brand-new turf field with seating for friends and family was estimated to be completed mid-year of the opening of the school in 2011.

The football team was a new team with kids from all over Brampton. There was only one team in the first year, which catered to 9th and 10th grade students. Since there was no turf, the future grizzlies had to practice about a mile from the school. Andrew and his new teammates would practice with a few coaches every weekday for August. When the summer came to an end, the practice would shorten. The athletes who passed all the conditioning would be awarded their uniforms and be a part of the first-ever football roster at

David Suzuki Secondary school. The first week of classes was everyone's first official week at the school. A three-story building with so much lighting, new faces, and brand-new athletic facilities. The school catered to a little over 500 students for the first year until the news broke about how great the resources were at the school. The first year Andrew had to play all of his games away because the football stadium was still developing. He would travel for almost 2 hours for some games on a school bus. Andrew knew those school bus trips were the best because he could crack jokes with his teammates, prepare for competition, and be a part of something for the greater good. That season was shaky; the team lost 4 games and won 3. Those 3 wins were crucial for developing the team's confidence in the program. If Andrew was not playing football for his city team or high school, he would be at the YMCA.

At 15, with his 16th birthday approaching, he was always trying to exercise. Even as a big kid, he had a lot of energy and would be running full-court games with 16, 17, and 18-year-old kids at the YMCA. These games were intense. One time Andrew got fouled, and his face was covered with blood. The ambulance came, and he had to get stitched up. Andrew embraced the intensity. He never complained or gave up on his effort and would bully some older kids on the court at times. The YMCA was in the heart of downtown Brampton. Beside the famous art theater, library nearby, train station to downtown Toronto and a diverse, rich culture in that area. Basketball was huge at the YMCA. The YMCA was like a church, somewhere where everyone was accepted and came to the common goal to compete and get in better shape. The YMCA had an indoor track, a weight room, a pool, a sauna, a yoga facility, and a basketball court. The YMCA worked with low-income families, treated disabled individuals like family, and never discriminated against anyone. Andrew felt comfort in the YMCA.

Andrew did not have many friends when he transferred from school to school and would mostly have a close relationship with athletes around the city. Andrew would get his conditioning from basketball and then go upstairs to get a workout. Exercising worked as therapy for Andrew's mental health. Andrew overcame his issues as a young child, and his misguidance was passed on from his father. Andrew got an annual membership which was cheap because he qualified for a low-income discount. Andrew would make sure his mom gave him some bus money so he could always be at the YMCA.

In the upcoming spring season, Andrew was finally at the legal age to work, and he began to look for jobs for the upcoming summer. The first job he got was working at the country's largest and most famous theme park, Canada's Wonderland. This theme park catered to world travelers and had hundreds of rides up to 400ft in the air. The job had employee discounts, free parking, and a fun atmosphere for high school students. Canada's Wonderland is an attraction for all ages. Located in Vaughan near the Grand shopping center Vaughan mills. Andrew failed the math test, so they put him as a groundskeeper and guide for guests for the season.

Andrew was upset at first, but then he changed his mind. He knew he needed income, and this situation would be able to help him have extra money. 10th grade was fast approaching, and he wanted to save up some money to pay for his team's uniform and buy some nice outfits for the fall term. Andrew worked 3-5 days every week. Andrew commuted from Brampton to Vaughan on a bus for 90 minutes before each shift and on the way back. Andrew enjoyed spending time with his new friends at work. His responsibility was to make sure the park was maintained, and he also was responsible for guiding tourists around the park. As the summer wound down and fall ball practice at his high school was fast approaching, Andrew felt excited about this year. Andrew was a sophomore and acquainted with Brampton, living there for 3 years now, where he was a part of a couple of teams, city and high school football. Andrew had some money saved from the summer and was excited about the future.

In the 10th grade, the turf field was complete, and it was time to compete for the varsity team. August was hot. It was a grind to practice on the turf and condition in the afternoons. Most players from last year came back to the program, and there were new additions. This summer, Andrew and his teammates were hitting 1-on-1s, Oklahoma drills, and a lot of collisions. At the end of the summer towards the beginning of the season and fall term, the Grizzlies were mentally prepared and physically. This season was something special. Andrew had more of a glow. He was beginning to attract many females and preparing for this season before and after practice. The turf field and the noise behind the team attracted many spectators at practice. This season was the first Friday night lights. Something really great for the community. The head coach had to purchase more bleachers because the fan base was growing fast. Andrew's best memories that season were the bus rides, the gate opening, and through a tunnel of cheerleaders on his way to take the field. That year Andrew was the starting nose tackle and offensive tackle.

Andrew could capitalize on his opportunities, and each week there was a college recruit at the game. Andrew was not educated much about college; he was not sure he would live to be 18 when he was in Toronto. At this point, he was just going with the flow. Andrew was dominant. He recorded sacks, opened a big hole for his small 5ft running back, and was overall physically gifted. At the age of 16, Andrew was 6'2 and 250 pounds. A good size for a defensive and offensive lineman at that age. The David Suzuki Grizzlies went 4-3 that year, an improvement from their first season record 3-4 and a more competitive schedule.

That year, there were awards given to outstanding athletes, and Andrew was given lineman of the year. He really should have won athlete of the year. Andrew played both sides of the football, was on special teams, and played 2 other sports that year: Basketball and rugby. In basketball, he played at the YMCA throughout high school with AAU players and college prospects. He also played basketball Thursday nights in Toronto when he was a troubled youth. Andrew felt that he had the capabilities to play for the team and became the starting center for the Jr team, which consisted of people from the 9th and 10th grades. You may say 6'2 is short to play center; however, at the age of 15 and 16, the tallest people in the city league were maybe 6'6, and all you had to do is make sure you got your rebounds and use your agility to get in front of the bigger players. Andrew recorded his first dunk that year. It's too bad it was at the YMCA and not an actual game.

There was a teacher's strike in the city of Brampton which canceled a lot of games; the tournaments still allowed the kids to play and get looks from college recruits. Rugby was a crazy sport 7 on 7 in the fall and 15 on 15 in the spring. Since Andrew was a part of the football team in the fall, he only played 15s in the spring. A real barbaric sport. Blood, injuries, and violence. The team was decent and traveled to face opponents across the city. This was the last year of Andrew being a multi-sport athlete. It was time to focus on the bread-and-butter sport American Football.

Andrew was invited to try out for the top 45 people in the province to be a part of Team Ontario. He made the tryouts and later traveled by plane back to Texas, near the place he played for Team Canada. That experience was eye-opening because the team had some good prospects and was competitive. It was coached by big-time university coaches and had a lot of sponsors that year. The opportunity was wonderful for Andrew and Kesha. Kesha was excited, helped pay for the trip, and would call to check up on Andrew while he was in Texas. Andrew was able to create his own playing card and compete against team USA again. This time the Canadians beat team USA 20-19 and flew back to Toronto late at night with a sense of pride and excitement.

The team was greeted by parents and loved ones with posters and signs showing support. The one person who was always there for Andrew was Kesha. Even though she was a single mother struggling to provide, she did her best. Kesha was involved, engaged, and supportive all throughout Andrew's life. Andrew's mom got sick and was frequently in the hospital. She would try to remain strong and keep her sickness hidden from Andrew. Her doctor recommended her medication to help improve her health. Andrew began to feel overwhelmed; he knew his mom was doing her best to make sure She was a part of the programs he was interested in, had a meal every day, and did whatever it took to keep the lights on in the apartment. Kesha was in a better situation living in Brampton because the violence was less; however, the apartment still was roach infested and was in a low-income neighborhood. Every morning, Kesha would make some breakfast for Andrew before she left for work. Andrew would take the city bus for 20 minutes toward his school. It became a routine. Family dinner was not a big thing in this household. The household felt empty at times to Andrew because he would make his own dinner and be in his room as hours passed until Kesha returned from her long shift.

Andrew transitioned from the theme park to working in the production department at Walmart. Andrew was the hardest worker, always on time, and always excited to learn new things. He was a vocal leader and always supported his coworkers. One day during the time he worked at his job, there was some jealousy because some of the managers would give Andrew more hours than his peers. One of the managers received a report that there were incidents of horseplaying with co-workers, and weekly, Andrew saw his hours beginning to shorten. Andrew eventually decided to leave that job. Andrew was unable to get into any relationships in high school. He found it difficult to love someone when no one has ever told him they love him. He would grab females' attention being a big-time football player in the city. Females would sit on his lap, grab his butt, and flirt with him. Andrew had no game, and he was heartless. He rarely showed love and let people in. He felt he had overcome so much and could not relate to people in Brampton who had big houses and spoiled their kids. Many people at this new school were middle class and above.

The students had their lives together and always talked about their parents' money to pay their college tuition. Andrew felt as if he could not fit in and felt like an outsider even though people looked up to him like a big brother. Ben, every couple of months, would contact his son and give Kesha a couple of hundred dollars to show his support as a father. When he would talk to his son, it would be to get everyone together to celebrate an event for him or his wife. One day, when Andrew had the weekend off from school, he was invited to go to his Dad's 6-bedroom house for his wife's birthday. His wife told her work friends that she's raised all of Ben's kids, and it was a big happy family. The interesting thing was that Andrew and his siblings would see each other about 20 days a year. This could be because Ben did not care to see his kids more or that he was too focused on painting a perfect family picture. It is difficult to portray a perfect family picture when you have 4 children by 4 different women; throughout that time, there was infidelity and an absence from the father. Ben was intelligent and made something out of himself as an immigrant.

There is only one issue with Ben: he was selfish, manipulative, and demeaning. Countless times when Andrew was younger, he would joke about Andrew's looks, shout at him out of aggression, verbally abuse him, and create an uncomfortable environment for all his kids. He would discourage his kids and be non-supportive in every dream, small or big. His constant disregard for his children was present throughout their childhood. Ask yourself this, would you be comfortable living in a mansion, eating really good, and your children live in poverty?

Andrew, now heading into his junior year of football and on the verge of turning 17 years old, you can see his work ethic has increased, and he is more engaged in the community. Andrew would volunteer at his grandma's church on the weekend and actively participate in church monthly. His grandma immigrated from Guyana and came to Canada with her mentally challenged son. She was a hard worker who had years in the medical industry and wanted to be close to her family. She lived with Andrew's aunt, who recently had twins. She was great for babysitting and home-cooked west Indian meals. Andrew began working harder and spending more hours at the YMCA training and outside playing football. The YMCA allowed Andrew to get bigger and stronger. He was now up 320 on the bench, 450 on the squat, and 560 on the deadlift. He put all life's obstacles into his workouts which allowed him to clear his mind and engage in something positive.

Andrew felt alone for most of his life. He felt as if his father might have taken away his confidence because of how he treated him, and this caused him to want to thrive and prove he was worth something. He was not the smartest person; he would be shy in class because he felt the other students were better than him. He would speak to his counselor Ms. Pouncy. Ms. Pouncy was probably the worst counselor for Andrew. She would look at his grades, consider Andrew a bad student, and recommend he step it up. She did not engage in effective ways for him to improve and did not show concern for his well being. When Andrew gained the confidence to ask questions, he finally asked one of the social science teachers if she could help him. Her response was everything was online as she proceeded to laugh with her work friends and head to lunch. The learning style at the school began to negatively impact Andrew more than be seen as beneficial to his progression. Andrew needed something different: a more close-knit environment where the teacher did not only care about reading off PowerPoints and getting paid. A few years later, Andrew was a senior. He had been working out all summer and had almost 5 years of development in football fundamentals, so the question was, "What's next?"

Andrew was a highly recruited athlete in Canada. By the age of 17, he had played 4 years as a starter for the Brampton Bulldogs, played for team Canada and team Ontario, and was among the top 60 all-Canadian football prospects. Andrew had recruits from almost every Canadian university football program and had a fair amount of D1-AA and junior college interest. He did not attend many events at his high school. He would skip the dances and athletic banquets, so he was not worried about skipping graduation. Andrew noticed everyone was planning which big university their parents would pay for or if they would jump straight into the workforce. Andrew knew he needed to decide quickly because graduation was a semester and a half away. Students were excited about Christmas break as November was fast approaching, and the fall term was almost over. Everyone at the school wanted gifts and to sit around the Christmas tree in their 5-bedroom big houses.

Andrew made the decision before Christmas break, he was going to prep school. Prep school is a private high school that caters to students from the 9th grade to the 12th grade. The curriculum is the same as a regular school with credible teachers. The school focuses on developing athletes who want to play college sports in Canada or the USA. The prep school was located an hour from the Buffalo, New York, border near a community college. It had a movie theater close by and several restaurants. Going to prep school for the spring of his senior year was eye-opening, and Andrew was exposed to different training routines for the next level. Throughout his time, one of his roommates was a future NFL third-rounder.

The facility was originally located in an old public school. When the facility moved, it had more of a large landscape. An indoor and outdoor practice facility, weight room, and class would be held on the second floor. Andrew had some of his best memories at the prep school. There was a lot of hitting in practice and good laughs among his teammates, and Andrew was even able to save his friend from getting arrested. One night, Andrew's friend Clay went to the grocery store around the corner from the hotel where the team stayed. Clay decided that it was a good night to shoplift. By doing that, he got caught and was taken into the back room by security.

The security told Clay the police were on their way. Clay asked for a phone call. Clay called Andrew, another football player, Smith, saying the police were on the way and he did not know what to do. If he called the head coach, he could get kicked out of prep school. The police told Clay he would get off on a warning; however, he needed to drop him off with his parents or guardian. Andrew was a great thinker, and he said to tell them, "You are a part of big brother, and I am your big brother." The funny thing was that it worked. The police drove around the corner with Andrew in the back to the hotel. Andrew and Smith waited anxiously outside the hotel, looking around and pacing themselves. They wanted to ensure that there was no sight of the head coach or owner of the school. The police finally decided to come out. Gun, taser, and baton on hip. Tall and assertive as the officer approached the players. The officer said, "Are you guys from Big Brother?" They replied, "Indeed, I am." The officer continued to explain the incident and that Clay was lucky to get off on a warning.

Andrew and Smith were quite large. They were 6'4 and 6'6 in height, so the officer believed they were part of big brother and said, "Here, you can take him." That night, Clay was lucky, and Andrew told him, "You needed to relax and make better choices." Prep school had a lot of issues going on. There was theft behind the scenes of the school. One of the partners of the school was caught pocketing the money. In the fall of 2015, Andrew was in his last semester of prep school. He was the starting right tackle and traveled to New York, Washington DC, and Ohio to play at some of the most competitive high schools in the USA. At the games, the coaches ranged from NAIA coaches to Power 5 scouts. Here came the downfall of Andrew's dream.

Andrew, after finishing high school and now working his way to be a college athlete, wanted to play on the highest level, which is division 1 football; it was not as easy as he had planned for it to be. Andrew always had a great work ethic. Andrew would stay late after practice and continue to condition on his off day, and the agility ladder was his best friend. His discipline gave Andrew the mindset of "I can play on the highest level."

He was convinced his time for success was at that moment, but was it? Andrew's time was winding down as it almost was December, and he knew he needed to speak to his advisor. His advisor was also the owner of the private school. He told him he wanted to get scouted by top universities in America and needed his help. Mr. Perkins pulled up Andrew's transcript and let him know it was not looking good. All of the years of struggling to have a voice in public school discussions put Andrew in a huge dilemma. Andrew took the ACT and scored a 19. His GPA was a 1.9 cumulative average. These academic credentials meant no Division 1 football. Andrew could not get a scholarship anywhere in the USA after prep school, which was a harsh reality. Andrew always heard stories of how the older generation who played football would be able to pay their way through school or the institution would cover up their academic deficiencies due to their outstanding athletic abilities. Andrew knew those were the old days, and in current society, you have to fight for what you want, or you will never reach your best outcome. At the age of 18, Andrew knew the people from his high school were headed to college and universities, and their future was set. He had left his graduation to go to prep school, and his grades did not match his talent.

On the verge of giving up and calling quits, he began to work to save up money. He moved from being a full-time truck unloader to an electrical wire cutter for clients. A couple months approaching his 19th birthday, he knew this industry was not for him. He was making 17$ an hour which was decent money for only having a high school diploma with no college experience. He knew another option could lead to division 1, which the head coach spoke to some players about. The coach was a former division 1 athlete, California-raised, all-American wide receiver coach Marlin. He was a great guy, an assertive leader, and had a history of having many connections in colleges and professional teams in North America. Marlin discussed junior college as a good route for Andrew. He said, "It won't be easy, but after 1-2 years, you can play your last 2-3 years in a big-time university." Andrew was broke. When I say broke, I mean Andrew took the bus every day and would barely be able to afford nice clothing. Andrew went into the bank with a little water, got a credit card, began to save some money from the factory, and began his training resume. Andrew would be around Canadian universities who would call him frequently with intentions for him to join their program. The coaches would show a lot of love.

One time, Andrew went on a visit to a university in downtown Toronto. He was escorted around by females, stayed at a hotel, ate a 5-star steak and lobster meal, and sat in a box suite looking down at the Raptors game in Toronto. The issue with the Canadian universities is they were offering 60% off of tuition, and you still had to pay for a meal plan and living expenses. Division 1 football programs paid for insurance, apartment, meal plans, and tuition. With refund checks and under-the-radar cash advances, a student-athlete could be bill free and still have up to 2000$ extra every month for necessities. The goal for Andrew was to go to junior college and then play division 1. These 2 were his short-term goals for the next few years. Andrew kept working hard on his craft and ensuring he was financially stable to move to California. As he continued working in the General labor and manufacturing industry, he was getting prepared to travel out before the end of August when the fall semester at the junior college was about to start, and football practice lifted off. Andrew was a social guy, big in stature and well-liked. He encountered a guy named Hamza.

Hamza was a business student and a family man who lived with his parents and a few siblings. Hamza would sometimes give Andrew rides when he took the bus after a long shift or invite him to hang out just to chill and pick up girls. However, Hamza had one more thing about him that made him a bad influence on Andrew. Hamza was a big-time drug dealer. Hamza would drive around selling drugs to mechanics, restaurant workers, anyone really. Hamza did not discriminate. Andrew had hung out with Hamza because his friends from high school had moved on with their lives, and he knew he was going a different path.

Hamza and Andrew would get women to have sex with them and always be the center of attraction. Andrew had the athletic build and looks, and Hamza would capture ladies with money. They were both great tag teams until it seemed like Hamza was bringing the negative out of Andrew and becoming a distraction. One night after a long day at work, Hamza invited Andrew to go out with him. Hamza said it would probably take an hour to commute, and there was a big show at a dance club near Niagara Falls. The legal age was 19. So, both men being around 19, thought it was a good time to make the most out of the night. Dressed to impress, the two men were. They had jeans on. Andrew wore a bright white t-shirt that had a crisp gold chain on his neck. Before Andrew went to the club, he went inside a trap house where Hamza's old investors stayed. Some people in that house were planning on being at the club later that night. Andrew and Hamza drove around the town. They got some food and then went to pick up one of Hamza's friends Rico.

Rico had been an ex-con with a lot of past charges under his name. Andrew immediately noticed when Rico came out of his apartment that he had a backpack that he threw in the trunk. Andrew – who had spent his childhood in a low-income neighborhood – knew that only trouble follows someone who has a backpack late at night and brings it wherever they go. More than likely, there is a weapon in it that can be used at the owner's discretion. This is where the story gets interesting.

Andrew, Hamza, and Rico pulled into the night club ready to have a great time and see how many numbers they could get. They passed through security. They got their jackets checked in and headed to their booth for the night. They drew attention because of the bottles coming to their section. Andrew and Hamza saw there were two thirsty females at the club, and they were looking for attention. The men started dancing with the women. They started getting really close, engaging in kissing and body rubbing. As the night finished, Andrew and Hamza were trying to continue their night with the females and proceeded to leave the club. There was only one issue.

The two females, thirsty for attention, had two boyfriends with whom they had come to the club with. Do you remember when I talked about Andrew and Hamza picking up a guy named Rico? Remember how he had a backpack that he put in the trunk? Rico was drinking in the background while the other men mingled with the females. They looked to the left as Andrew and Hamza proceeded outside the nightclub. It was dark outside. It was after 2 AM; naturally, no cars were driving in sight. Everyone was either in the club or at home. As the men turned their bodies, they saw Rico surrounded by two men.

The females were still with Andrew and Hamza when they told them the men around Rico were their boyfriends. There was a verbal exchange expressing to Rico that they had their girlfriends in the trunk the entire night. Andrew and Hamza could feel the tension in the air. The men tried to intimidate Rico even though he had been drinking the entire night. Hamza waited by the car, but Andrew felt he needed to step in. Andrew had always been a person with values and someone who always felt like a protector. So, Andrew came into the mix. He drew his brass knuckles. Rico reached in his backpack and pulled out his pistol. Shots were fired, but no one got hurt, and the men left with their girlfriends. Andrew, Hamza, and Rico hopped in the Audi and left the area.

Andrew and Hamza dropped Rico back at his apartment and then hopped on the highway on their way back to Brampton. This was one of the examples of how Hamza became a bad influence on Andrew. Andrew could have got caught up in Canada and lost his opportunity to play college football in the United States. This incident happened a month before he had to fly out to junior college. Instead, Andrew continued working out and trying to balance his full-time job schedule. As the summer was coming to an end, it was July and time to say goodbye to his friends and family. Andrew made his way around town and decided to pay his father a visit.

Ben would not be supportive, angry at him as if he was jealous of his opportunity. Before leaving his weekend stay, he told Andrew, "Make sure you do not come back a disappointment." Andrew did not know how to take that and was expecting a more supportive time with his Dad, and he would have loved to hear he would be a part of his journey throughout college. Well, Andrew did not get that. There was no indication his father would speak to him throughout his college time. Andrew knew it was time to get focused on the goal of playing Division 1 football. He needed to cut off all negativity and distractions. Hamza, the drug dealer, had to go. Non-supportive, verbally abusive father had to go. It was as simple as that.

If there are negative people in your life, whether it is family or friends, and you have tried to make it a positive experience, but it keeps on being negative, it is time to move forward with positive people. The closest people in your life may not want you to succeed. Trust the people that want the best for you, and there are more positive experiences with them than negative. Here is a breakdown of positive people and negative people. If they are negative, remove them completely after the 3rd time they show they are negative until they can prove you differently long term. That might sound harsh, but it is necessary.

Positive is a person who does something selfless, a person who is engaged with their family and friends, and a person who is empathetic and has good core values. A negative person is someone who does something for the betterment of themselves, a person who has better resources and would look down on someone less fortunate, and a person who creates an uncomfortable situation.

Andrew began packing his suitcase, made sure he had sent in all his paperwork to the community college, and broke the ties with his employer 2 weeks before flying out. The one thing Andrew knew he was going to miss was his favorite Caribbean food spots. His favorite spot that was close by was Sunrise Jamaican Cuisine. It was located near the YMCA, where he worked in the center of Downtown Brampton. Andrew called the junior college he committed to in Kansas and found out right before he wanted to go to school days before departure that the junior college was not interested in Andrew's talent. The school felt he was an average prospect out of high school and had a mediocre film out of prep school. Andrew was worried at this point. He was unable to qualify for a division 1 scholarship. He already closed the door on all Canadian universities. Andrew was uninterested in playing in Canada; he did not respect how much financial aid was given to the student-athletes and wanted to play against the best competition at the college level.

Thanks to luck and hard work, he had found another coach who was interested in rebuilding his team from years past. This program resided in the desert, a small city named Victorville in California, 3 hours from Los Angeles. The bald-headed coach had over 30 years of experience in college football. He was tied to junior colleges all over the country, peaking in division 1 as a coach; he now ran a good football program that had been a championship team for many years. The program was the cheapest junior college in California. It would run Andrew about 30,000 for tuition and board for 2 years of his 5 years of college eligibility. Andrew made sure he had whatever loans, credit cards, and savings accounts accessible before he said goodbye to his family. Andrew did not know if he would be a starter at the community college. He did not know if he would have enough talent to play after junior college. He did not even know if he had enough financial support to afford college without a scholarship. One thing about Andrew was that he was self-motivated, intrigued by the opportunity, and had an incredible ability to adapt.

The week before summer training camp Andrew had to get everything ready. He hustled to get his paperwork in order with the community college guidance counselor and emphasized his commitment to the coaching staff. The interest that was shown allowed Andrew to feel a sense of fulfillment and know he was making a great choice for his future.

Early in August, 3 weeks before the fall semester started, it was time for training camp at Victor Valley Community College. Humid, dusty, and old was the best way to describe the high desert and the Inland Empire. When Andrew arrived at the airport, he was greeted by his head coach. He picked him up in an old truck, you could tell he had a big personality, and they both had great respect for each other. It was a great start to a player and coach relationship. They drove about 90 minutes from the airport. There was little traffic, so it was smooth sailing to the college.

The college briefly toured before arriving at the off-campus apartment to meet some of his roommates who were a part of the 2016 Victor Valley College roster. The college was old and had a lot of potholes in the grass-based field. The college did not play on the grass field and instead played at a local high school. Which was interesting and motivating for Andrew at the same time. It was important for Andrew to get adjusted to his surroundings since he would commit to the program for the next 2 years with the goal of earning his associate's degree.

They eventually transitioned to the house where he stayed and met his teammates. The house was diverse; it included some players from Hawaii, New York, and Texas. Everyone was excited. The season was a month away, and training camp began in a few days. The young men mingled and got to know each other, and everyone got situated in the rooms. It was a good dynamic in the 5 bedroom, 2 full restrooms, a large backyard, and a big living room house. The only problem was the transportation. Uber was a growing company at the time, and the bus trip would take 90 minutes to commute to the college on average once you walked 20 minutes to the station and waited another 20 minutes. There were some funny characters in the group, especially the Hawaiian brothers. They were 2 strong men with long hair touching their backs. They were always singing and would have freestyle battles amongst themselves. They were a joy to be around, and they would commute to the college every day with

Andrew. Passing many houses, as they made a left from the house they lived at, they continued towards the bus station.

The bus station was busy on a Tuesday afternoon in the middle of training camp. The classrooms were still closed as the semester start date approached. The athletes for the football team would meet together in portables and get to know each other. The head coach would speak to the team and let them know what the goals are for the season and how he wants the team to achieve them. The head coach had a lot of wisdom and was respected. He was a funny and relatable man; he always made sure to keep it real with his players. The team was filled with a lot of different backgrounds – European, Hawaiian, and African. People came from all over the United States, many from the west coast since the college was in California.

The team was ready to build on the championship culture. Victor valley college was back-to-back champions in 2014 and 2015. Coming together as a team was extremely important for the team they were close to. The team had been filled with athletes who played against each other and competed in tough games in the championship years; therefore, it was easier for the team to be able to transition into a new year with incoming players. The team itinerary during the summer would include a workout and 3 hours of practice on the field Monday through Friday. Throughout those days, there would be positional meetings which are when offense and defense have meetings to discuss the upcoming schedule and what needs to be done as a football program to enhance peak performance. Andrew was able to feel out the environment, and he always was quick on his feet. Andrew was an athlete, 6'4, 280 pounds, with good posture and a great build for an NFL offensive lineman. He was physical and violent. He had a lot of passion for the sport and was committed to working on his fundamentals. People were sometimes intimidated by his confidence and strength.

Andrew was putting up ridiculous numbers at the age of 19. Squatting 600 pounds, benching 400 pounds, and deadlifting 700 pounds. Andrew trained so hard he would go to practice sore and with muscle inflammation. He did not care; he was the strongest in the room and the best offensive lineman on the team. Andrew was coached well and eager for the first game. After that, every day at practice was constant competition. There were some great players this year. There was a lot of explosion, speed, and power within the team.

Fast forward to the first game, the season opener; you could hear the noise from the stadium. It was a home game. Everyone was getting taped up and was ready for competition. It was a warm Saturday at Silverado high school, and it was time to go. Everyone was padded up and knew it was time to have a competitive game. Andrew came out of the locker room, walked onto the field, and knew it was time. The lights were bright, the fans were excited, and the team repeated their team chant. Andrew, before the game, liked to sit on the bench and reflect on his journey. He began thinking about his mom struggling to pay rent, and his Paps, who never cared if he made it home or not. He thought about his physical abuse when he was young. From that point on, he knew he was not afraid anymore. He was not afraid of death. He made up his mind he was willing to die on the field for a chance to get a division 1 scholarship. Andrew was ready to play every snap like his last. The quarterback would yell out "10!" "10!" "Hut!" After the snap cadence, it was go-time.

The offensive line was the most difficult position on the field. These men were protectors for the rest of the offense, and with one missed step, the play could be turned over. For instance, there were 5 offensive linemen, but sometimes, there may have been an extra offensive lineman who was lined up to the tackle. He probably would have had to check in as a weak side or strong side tight end. As Andrew took his first snap, he ensured his elbows were tucked in, pad level low, and punched his opponent. Andrew would punch the defender's chest so hard that he immediately fell on his back. Andrew made sure to take the soul out of the defender's body, opening up the play for the running back, which led to a touchdown. The bleachers were packed, and it was loud; the entire community was out. It was the end of the summer, and everyone was getting ready for the fall. The football game created a great atmosphere for families to come and interact with each other. There was a concession stand that sold snacks and drinks. There also was a great cook who made sure to throw down a great meal for the attendees. Many of the players and families after the game would stay back and get a meal from the concession stands. Unfortunately, this game did not end as well as planned. After the rams got the win, there was a fight in the parking lot. Many players from both teams were involved in the altercation. This was the result of the ass whopping the away team received.

There were players getting body slammed on cars, punches to the face, and a scene of chaos. It was crucial that there was someone that came to break up the dispute and ensure that the league's reputation was not tarnished during the incident. The incident created despair and anxiety amongst everyone at the game. Luckily, Andrew could leave the scene and go home with one of his buddies, Aron. Aron was a man of good character and a reliable teammate. Aron and Andrew often commuted from their apartment complex to the college. They were both offensive linemen, so their bond grew tighter as the season progressed. Finally, the night came to a close.

The members of each team who were involved in the incident were separated and proceeded to leave the stadium shortly after. The stadium lights turned off. Game 1 was in the books. Sunday was a day for recovery and injury prevention treatment with the athletic trainer, which is usually the itinerary for most college football programs in the United States. This game was a transition to the beginning of the fall semester. The semester began on Monday.

Every athlete had an athlete contract that must have been signed and upheld throughout their commitment to the football program. Each athlete must commit to holding up a good GPA, being a good role model, avoiding substance abuse, and showing they were an asset instead of a liability to the program. Let's talk about assets and liabilities.

These are two key principles that many of us stood on for our core values of the people we accepted in our lives. An asset is someone that brings something positive and is an influential part of our lives. A liability is someone that is negative, usually jealous, or does not care about your growth. Ask yourself, would you rather have assets or liabilities in your life? When you come up with the answer, check who is an asset, who is a liability, and immediately remove the liabilities from your life – regardless of them being old acquaintances, friends, or family members. Know that liabilities are what they are... liabilities.

It finally turned Monday, the start of a new semester. Everyone had their best fits on, the sun was shining down on campus, and there were events throughout the facilities. Many students had to get their id cards for the year, and it was a good day to be on campus and get involved in the student activities. Team meetings were scheduled for 1 PM, and positional meetings were set for 2 PM. There was a news article headlined in the local paper about the Rams football team. Within the article, the altercation that took place late Saturday evening and the season opener was highlighted on the front page. Anyone that read the entire article could see that the team was getting a bad reputation, and there might be penalties moving forward.

Now it was time for the team meeting. The first day of class was on Monday at 1 PM, and everyone met in the big portable near the coaching office; it was emphasized not to be late. The team headed in. They were excited to celebrate the win and a new fall semester was a breath of fresh air for the team. For the coaches, it was not the same outlook. The coaches had something else in mind. The coaches did not only feel embarrassed, but they felt as if the team did not hold up the athletic contract they signed and they were bringing a bad reputation to the program. The college president had to call the head coach and figure out what went wrong and how the incident could be prevented. The coach felt he was in a vulnerable position, and now his job coaching these men may be in jeopardy. The head coach had no choice but to get upset at his team. His message can be summarized by his preaching that it was immature and ruined the program's integrity. He also emphasized that there will be police officers from that point on to ensure the safety of the people at each game is prioritized. The team was not mad at the coach for speaking his mind. The coach also showed that he was proud of the team for having each other's backs that day. Even though the college does not support physical violence, it was good for the coaching staff to see unity, and this might allow the team to be more cohesive throughout the season.

Andrew left the meeting and went to sit with some of his offensive lineman friends in the coaching offices. It was almost time for positional meetings to start, and it was time to break down the film for the game. The film session was always a good time for Andrew. He could be with his teammates and rank up who had the most pancake blocks each game.

Another bonus is there was a lot of joking around with the men. As the semester progressed, the games accumulated in the 10-game schedule. The Rams had a decent record; they were 3-2 and looking for the beginning of conference play in a few weeks. The Rams had some dynamic players, from running backs to explosive defensive linemen. It was an elite-level roster and a great time for everyone to be engaged in the program.

On a Saturday night, Andrew and some of his roommates at their house on Tonawanda Rd in Apple Valley decided to throw a house party and charge an entry fee. The house had 5 bedrooms, so there was a lot of space and room for students and locals who wanted to come to the party. The party went well, and there was a lot of money being made among the roommates. A few hours in, a small car pulled into the driveway. Struggling to get out of the car, there was a 400-pound man with some chew in his mouth. It was coach Carson. Coach Carson was not only the offensive lineman coach for the program but also lived a few blocks away from the house in Apple Valley. Carson came to the door where Andrew was accepting the entry fee for the house party, smelling like a donut and cigarettes. Andrew was surprised that coach Carson was up that late.

Coach Carson told Andrew he had just passed the house on his usual fast-food run and the party was so loud and had so many cars it drew a lot of attention from the neighborhood. Andrew was surprised to see coach Carson and he let him into the house. When the coach entered, it smelled like a bar, a dispensary, and a strip club. The house was packed. The issue was that many people consuming substances were not guaranteed they were all legal, and that was a major red flag. Coach Carson rounded up all the players at the house and ensured they were not under the influence since they were all mostly under 21 and as they were the responsibility of the football coaching staff. The main priority for the coach was to ensure the safety of the players and protect the house since it was being rented for the academic calendar year. The players disbursed once they saw the coach and then migrated back together after some persuasion from Andrew. Andrew made sure to keep the peace at the party when all of the commotions were going on with the coach and the players. Some people did not want to leave, but they had to go. Eventually, everyone left the house, and there was no overwhelming issue. Coach Carson emphasized the importance of being positive role models and protecting the program's integrity. He also noted that there would be consequences. Monday could not have come any faster. Andrew and his teammates felt the weekend went by quickly after Saturday night's party.

Now, it was Monday. It was a fresh week. 4 days of practice, travel day, and then game day Saturday, an away game. A couple hours' drive outside the desert. Monday at practice, it was right when the sun was at its peak. 100 degrees that day, 3 PM, everyone apart from the football program had to get dressed and head out to the practice facility. I failed to mention that the practice field had large hills next to it, so it was a great place to get conditioning done. The hills were the player's worst nightmare, especially after they finished competing with each other. It seemed like an exhausting task. Well, it was the Tonawanda's houses' lucky day. The roommates and teammates had the pleasure of going up that hill. The head coach told them in the middle of practice after the players had been competing for some time. He specified the players had hill runs for the remainder of practice because they wanted to throw a party and serve to an underage audience. Reminder: there would still be an hour and a half remaining before practice ends. Some players decided to go home and believed it was an unfair punishment, some players began running up the hill, and some started cursing at the coach. Eventually, practice went on, and the coach allowed the players who remained on the hill to stop about 30 minutes into the hill runs. Andrew was one of the men who stayed. They were in the middle of 1-on-1s, Andrew's favorite drill.

1-on-1 is when the offense and defense go against each other. Within lineman 1-on-1s, there is not much playing around. This is as physical as it gets on the football field. The team's biggest and baddest individuals play on the offense and defense line. A quick breakdown of how 1-on-1s go amongst linemen is the defensive line would line up in the gap in front of the offensive lineman. Then, depending on the snap account, the offensive lineman would move off that cadence and is responsible for locking up the opposing defensive lineman. This drill is crucial to the flow of each football game. The lineman controls the game's pace as much as the quarterback does. If you ever watch a football game, it does not matter if it is pewee or the pros. Take a minute to look at people in front of the quarterback. These are the people constantly fighting for position and protecting the quarterback at all costs. With one missed step from an offensive lineman, the play is over. If you have ever watched a team lose a football game at a high level, it is probably because of a lack of protection for the quarterback or running back or a lack of penetration from the defensive line to the quarterback. Having practice simulations of games is crucial for growing programs and building the fundamentals of technique over power training.

Power training is important in the off-season, but it is not the most important. Power training should be valued as much as conditioning is and should not be overvalued at any time. Football is a physical sport; therefore, it is important to develop your muscle strength and ensure you have great body control. The importance of technique and fundamentals is what the Rams football program stood for and enlightened the team on how to enhance body performance and recovery. Within 1-on-1s, constant hand fighting for leverage, certain body angles, and flexibility are required to play offensive linemen. To be an offensive lineman, you must commit to pain, hard work, and no excuses. All you do is hit. Every play, every drill, and every day during a season. You are expected to physically remove a grown man repeatedly who is over 6 ft and weighs more than 260 pounds. It is a position that stems from mental toughness, and it is a great asset when building character and willpower. Without offensive lineman, no holes are being opened up in games, and there are no 50-yard touchdowns by quarterbacks. Being an offensive lineman can age your body quickly; it is difficult to stay still or have little motion when there is a 300-pound man constantly trying to get past you and hit your quarterback. Andrew's 1-on-1s were usually a DOA for the opposition.

Andrew had the strongest punch on the team and was ready to embarrass his competition. His technique was nearly perfect. His coach taught him well and used his learning to enhance his performance. As much as Andrew was a player on the field, he was a player off the field. Andrew was a big, strong, and agile athlete. He was respected on campus and had a lot of female attention. His teammates admired his wisdom and experience from prep school to being a college sophomore. Offers began to come in, Andrew was more focused, and his GPA was on the right track to earning him a full division 1 scholarship. Andrew got offers from Arkansas State, Louisiana Lafayette, Cincinnati, San Diego State, and others. The university coaches would call his junior college head coach and tell him they admired his physicalness for the game and would like to arrange an official visit. Andrew continued to work hard in the gym, improving his posture and becoming more confident.

# PART 2

–

# DOWNFALL AND FAILURE

With everything good, there is always a twist. A failure is a negative experience you cannot control that is not intentional.

With all the offers that Andrew received, he attended a few visits. He went to San Diego State, partied like a rockstar, and had some of his best memories of that visit. Andrew went with some of his friends. The school was near a beach. The beach had a beautiful atmosphere. There were a lot of people from all over the world to see the beautiful body of water. Around the beach, there were many restaurants where locals could meet and greet. The school itself had a beautiful modern look as it accommodated a large body of students. The stadium was huge, and there were many awards to show the great culture of the institution. When Andrew visited the university, he felt like he was in a movie.

He never would have imagined being able to go to such a big-time university, but the opportunity presented itself. The parties were legendary around the school, especially after a football game. Fancy cars, beautiful women, what else can a student want? A student that attended that university for undergraduate or graduate studies would be able to have the time of their life. When Andrew and some of his friends entered one of the parties, everyone was in tune with the music and knew it would be a great time. Andrew had many similar opportunities to go to universities like this and have a visit.

He continued the season, and as it dwindled down to the last 4 games, he was trying to plan out his future and spoke to his advisor about transferring to a different program. He wanted to get a breakdown of his athletic eligibility. When Andrew discussed his education plan that was created a little over a year back when arriving in California, he was told he would be able to complete his coursework and finish his 2 seasons of junior college achieving his associate's degree in 3 semesters. Well, this was not the case. In Andrew's updated advising session, he heard other news.

See, at the beginning of this section, I discussed, "With everything good, there is always a twist." Well, this phrase soon became a reality for Andrew. Andrew, after high school, played one year of private school football and 2 seasons of junior college football; therefore, he should have been left with 3 years of eligibility when transferring to a division football program. It all sounded good when Andrew arrived on campus. Still, the education plan was altered and ultimately caused a dilemma in Andrew's progression towards graduating and transferring to an FBS program. The advisor at the college informed Andrew that he would only be eligible for 3 years at d1 if he completed an additional semester with 6 classes in the spring to graduate. The education plan was all screwed up.

The education plan initially was not altered around, and it was more than reasonable for Andrew and his mom. He knew he did not have the money. Coming from a low-class family and living rent to rent, it was difficult to pay bills. Without a scholarship or any additional support, there was no way he could graduate college. His credit card was maxed out, and he only had a few dollars left to his name. Faced with a decision to go back to Canada to work and try to balance the classes online or not graduate college and lose all his FBS offers that he had worked so hard for years and years on end. Since Andrew was on a student visa, he could only work certain hours, which had to be a part of his major. He could not get last-minute employment, and it seemed as if it was a repeating pattern that every time Andrew completed his football season, the coaches would move on to recruiting other prospective athletes. Their focus would shift from the previous athletes.

The best coaches in the world are those who could relate to the player and find time to make sure a prospect is financially and mentally comfortable. With this methodology, an athlete can perform to his or her peak performance. Andrew was out of options. Coaches moved on quicker to a new prospect than a dog chasing a cat. One thing that Andrew's junior college coach told him was coaches at the higher college levels were cowards. They would show interest and then could leave you on read as soon as another eligible prospect became available. These coaches would not give you notice; they would not care about your work ethic; it's mostly about size and eligibility. Size and eligibility were two of the most important factors when attending an FBS school.

In this division, they looked for freaks to fill in positions of weakness during the season from past mistakes. In terms of eligibility, they looked for academically and athletically eligible people. In academics, typically, you needed a 2.0 GPA to be eligible; however, a 3.0 or above landed more opportunities. Athletically, there were usually 5 years of eligibility in college, and you could play all those years. Many student-athletes used up 4 years in a sport and left 1 year in case they did not want to play that year or 1 year in case they were injured. These 2 instances were called a red shirt and a medical red shirt.

As the end of October was fast approaching in the fall of 2017, the students at the college began getting ready for finals and presentations. Graduation and the end of the fall term was fast approaching. Everyone who was not taking any winter classes would be off for over a month for winter break.

Andrew could not process a loan application, had no money left and exhausted all options.

He contacted his absent father to see if he could assist with any financial support. He even promised to pay back everything. Ben had other priorities; this, unfortunately, was not one of them. That made Andrew angry but hungry. He knew his dream of playing at a big-time FBS school was diminishing, and he had to focus on what to do next to overcome this obstacle and still have a chance of playing football at a high level in America. Andrew had an intense workout that day. Working out had always been therapy for Andrew. Strength and conditioning had been the healthiest way for Andrew to clear his mind and get through any mental issues he faced. Andrew's grades were good for the fall term, so he was not worried about finishing the semester strong. Andrew's concern was his eligibility and lost offers.

After the semester ended, he returned to Canada and got a full-time job unloading trucks. Various name brands were required to be shipped and stocked at the job. The job paid decently, and it was a good job that he could work immediately. Andrew attempted to balance his 40 hours trying to pay for school while he had to take 6 classes to graduate in the spring at Victor Valley College. He was about a month into taking his classes when he was emailed by the college president. The president needed to verify his enrollment since he was an international student, which was a normal annual procedure. This procedure could take place in that fall or the spring semester depending on the enrollment at the college. She indicated that Andrew had fled the country, and his visa was revoked. She proceeded to drop all of his 6 classes and refunded any initial payment made towards his coursework at the college.

What now? This was the question that surrounded Andrew. He was lost, he thought he had everything going for him, and it looked like he had nothing going for him now. Andrew's mom moved him from the violence in Toronto. He began playing football and developed into a great athlete in junior college. Well, at this point, it felt like the end of his journey. Only a high school degree, athletic eligibility diminishing, and no scholarship. Andrew was finally out of options and was getting depressed. There is a quote that a lot of people liked to say hard work beats talent when talent doesn't work hard. The people that said that quote probably are not talented. The quote was a general statement with no specific meaning. You did not have to work hard if you were talented or had accumulated assets. This statement was a fact. Suppose you inherited a fortune or had gifted abilities, either intellectually or athletically. In that case, your effort could be minimal, and you would still achieve the same outcome against someone who had worked hard their entire life. The one thing about Andrew was that he knew he would find a way.

He turned his back on Canadian university football; his mindset was d1 or bust. His goal was not to play professional football at this point but to reach his dreams of being a division 1 football player. He wanted to sit with the most highly ranked players in college football before his eligibility was over. This was when it got hard; Andrew needed to finish these classes in person in California to finish a college degree. Andrew was working full-time and thousands of miles away. His only support system was his mom who could not afford to send him to college. He needed to make a path on his own. Faced with this challenge, Andrew worked like a slave every day in the peak heat of the spring and summer. Andrew never had a car, so he would have to commute on the city bus an hour on average to and back from any destination. He worked 2 jobs when there was availability; the jobs all were general labor and factory manufacturing careers.

The jobs required you to constantly lift over 60 pounds. At times, you may have to unload a truck of 400 60-pound boxes by yourself. People would complain about back issues and pain, but that did not make the job easier. A business is a business. A business is about production, so if you were not performing, they would find someone to replace you. In most general labor positions in the GTA (greater Toronto area), there were warehouses that housed employees and had an evaluation scale. This scale usually had 2 differences in how the employees were evaluated. When a new hire came in, they started off as a temporary Associate with the possibility of moving up to a definite position. The secure position that many people wanted in these jobs was full-time. With full time you had more freedom and benefits that were accessible. In many of these temporary to full-time positions, there was a trend of immigrants, green card visa holders, and elders that worked in these establishments. The people working at these places believed the dream was to work hard and achieve full-time status. Whoever had worked in different careers understood there was always an evaluation or an opportunity to move up in a company. The people that achieved this level of power had to kiss ass. No one had ever moved up in a company without kissing ass unless their success was due to inheritance.

Andrew was not looking for a full-time position with benefits, he just needed constant income and he knew he was going to get as much money saved up as possible throughout the spring and summer. He made sure he was a leader, always on time, and most importantly, made sure he did the job right every time. This foundation was a learning tool for his success later on. The calls still came in. Andrew's junior college film was one of the best in the country for offensive line, and he had good size for the position. Andrew had almost 20 division 1 schools interested in giving him a full scholarship. One coach at Cincinnati even told him that the players stayed in high-rise condos and he would be able to get a penthouse suite. As a young athlete, that could be a gift and a curse. Andrew liked to stay humble. Andrew was determined, and as hard as he worked in the warehouse, he dedicated his time to strength and conditioning and treatment for any past injuries at a local sports clinic. Andrew had some work to do; he now had 6 classes that had to be taken in the fall. He needed to save every penny from the spring and summer to afford those classes on campus and pay rent for an apartment near the college. Junior colleges did not typically accommodate international students, so everything he made was typically out-of-pocket expenses. Football and academics became girlfriends 1 and 2 in Andrew's life.

Andrew was not playing with his future anymore. He refused to participate in anything that would not develop his skills on the field or make him money. He used to be the life of the party but not anymore; he did not even think about having fun. The last 3 parties he attended in California ended badly. The first one ended with a shootout and multiple people getting into a physical altercation, and the second one ended with someone getting stabbed in front of him and someone getting beat up by multiple gang members. In the last party, he recalled a shooting, and everyone stormed inside. Andrew and one of his teammates in junior college from Florida had to stay hidden in the restroom until the party settled. The point is that fun comes with consequences, and Andrew refused to keep playing with his future. He was now an all-conference offensive lineman, heavily recruited in the United States, and his name traveled through football coaching offices. He knew he needed focus and discipline if he wanted to make something positive out of his challenging situation. Even though the situation may have been challenging, it was not overwhelming. Andrew believed that everything great in life is attainable with time and effort; he had that kind of an outlook.

Eligibility is something that is not taught enough to young athletes by coaches and faculty at a public or private school. A typical student transitioning to college from secondary school usually only needs to focus on their grades and their aptitude testing (or SAT) scores when attending an academic institution in the United States. When considering a potential prospective student who wanted to attend college and had athletic talent and academic competence, it was essential to help them understand their options at least by their sophomore year in high school. The reason there should be some level of competence before they entered their junior year was to give them 1-2 years to get future goals in order and ensure they were on the right track. This responsibility could be left to a student; however, parents needed to put in more effort to be involved in their children's success in high school. In high school, many students went through a lot of growing pains as they developed into their roles as adults. In high school, there had been many instances of counselors and teachers not building up a student's confidence, not enabling them to have the resources they needed to reach their full potential. This could be due to a lack of salaries which causes a lack of interest beyond a lesson plan.

What Andrew found out later on in his life was that college was more manageable than high school. Could this be because college-level learning is less than high school? This could not be the answer that would not academically make sense. The reason is that there are more resources available. You have to pay for those resources; however, those resources on any given campus can enhance a student's performance tremendously. High schools have limited resources, and the lack of caring from many teachers in the public school system is troubling and discouraging. Is it possible for a student to have a 1.9 GPA in high school and earn a 3.75 GPA in university? Well, anything is possible with a mentality of being consistent and never being satisfied. Now let's go back and discuss Andrew's circumstances.

He was currently in Canada, saving up money to head back to California in August to complete his last semester. This entire process had pushed his graduation back 2 terms. Spring and summer had passed, and Andrew was forced to return to Canada because of visa status issues, and he needed to work to pay for tuition and board. If Andrew had been able to complete his associate degree in the spring, which he planned to, he would have been able to be on a division 1 football field at the beginning of summer. This would have given him plenty of time to learn the playbook and get in peak shape for the upcoming game 1 kick-off for the season in late august. Andrew also would have 3 years of eligibility which could be all used, or he could have 1 year to learn the system of a prospective football program and still have 2 years remaining of eligibility for on-field performance. Plans altered; this was when Andrew got to his low point, and his entire perspective of his outcome in college needed to be adjusted. Since Andrew's new plans were to graduate after the upcoming fall semester after he returned on a new i-20 visa reissued by the president.

Once universities began understanding the situation, they started to backtrack. The interest and offers once were there no longer existed no longer. Andrew was messed up mentally more than anything. He was bussing his ass for years and felt that the outcome would be him going to a big-time division 1 program. Now he felt overwhelmed. He was at a shaky point in his life; he did not have many friends since he chose to attend college in the United States. Many of his closest friends and people he mingled with when he moved to Brampton moved on either with relationships, or they were at some university in Canada on or off campus. People always like to say the phrase "to nothing comes easy." The only question about this phrase is, "When do blood, sweat, and tears result in success? How long does a person have to do the right thing and struggle before they achieve?

Well, this is what Andrew constantly asked himself not only at his lowest point of college but when he was willing to die on the field on game day, which led him to all of those FBS division offers. If plan B all went as planned, Andrew would have been able to graduate with his associate of art degree at the end of the fall semester and transfer to division 1 in the spring of 2018. This would have allowed him to train with his new team in the spring and summer, giving him plenty of time to be ready for competition. Andrew would still have 2 years of eligibility at division 1. Will everything go as planned the second time around? We will have to see.

It is hard to stay focused in a time filled with challenges, but it's possible. As simple as that statement is, it is because you have the power to change any situation. You only lose the ability to change a situation when you give up. When you quit, it shows that you are weak and lack willpower. If you want to overcome a difficult challenge, try to think of the process instead of the outcome and see how that mentally allows you to be more attentive to the task at hand.

Andrew began to lose passion for the sport of football. His mentality was backward; he was so focused on attending a big-time college that he failed to acknowledge the process of getting there. His mindset was determined, willing to learn, and always ready to adapt, but did that bring him to where he needed to be? The answer is absolutely not. Something needed to change if Andrew wanted a successful outcome and not be a college dropout. He had to think really hard about what he needed to accomplish and how much his mom struggled to ensure she kept him on the right track when he was a child.

Andrew decided he was going to fly out of Toronto in late August. Andrew said goodbye to his family. He knew there was a good chance he would not be able to come to visit them until Christmas. He packed his large suitcase the night before he was scheduled to depart. He made sure to weigh it, he did not want to pay any oversize fees, and wanted a smooth check-in. The next morning, he called for a ride to the airport. The ride was about a 20-minute commute to the airport from his apartment in Brampton.

The flight was smooth, but there was a layover; he had to wait a long time for his final flight to Ontario, California.

The head coach had a relationship with Andrew. They were together for 2 years and lost by one touchdown in the conference finals in Andrew's freshman year. Their bond was good because Andrew needed housing for the fall, and he could be accommodated a few weeks before arriving. Andrew was not aware of where he would be able to stay for the 16 weeks; however, he did not care; he was grateful for the opportunity. Housing is something that can take months to get depending on what city and state. Andrew arrived at the airport and had one of his friends from past seasons pick him up. They both headed to the coaching office.

The coaches were in the middle of fall camp since it was late August when Andrew arrived. Andrew went to the field after being notified. Andrew came out in sunglasses, a Versace chain, and a green polo. You already knew he was ready for the spotlight. Andrew proceeded to greet his coach and some of his former teammates. He also made sure to interact with roommates for the semester. His roommates were at the time on the practice field finishing their workout.

After practice, Andrew greeted the head coach, met up with the head coach, and updated his plans for the future. Andrew put his luggage in his roommate's car and headed to his apartment for the semester. On the way, you could see many restaurants and students in the area. Andrew was not involved in fall camp this year, so when he came to the college, it was right before the school year started. It was weird for him to be at the college and only focus on coursework. In years past, he would be getting ready for game 1 of the season in late August.

The arrangement for the semester was not the best; when Andrew arrived at his apartment, there were 3 bedrooms and 1 restroom. The 3 bedrooms had 2 roommates, and there were 6 people throughout the rooms. Andrew had two options for his last semester: sleep on an air mattress on the floor or find somewhere else to sleep. Out of options and in need of graduating at the end of the fall semester, he accepted the arrangements and made the air mattress his bed for the semester. The issue with sleeping in the living room was that there were many people in and out of the house, there was a lot of noise that you couldn't avoid, and if you had classes in the morning, you may be kept up by roommates because you stayed in the living room. It was pretty much an unavoidable situation for Andrew in this circumstance.

The area where Andrew stayed was the ghetto – full of crackheads, gang bangers, and low-income housing. The housing was in Victorville, a 15-minute bus ride once you walked 10 minutes to the bus stop and a 5-minute smooth drive when you passed the convenience store down the street on the corner of the block. It was the start of class, and Andrew got his schedule from the school's online database and proceeded to get acquainted with his surroundings. Andrew completed 3 semesters at the college; therefore, it did not take him long to find his landmarks. After he got settled in, he went to the cafeteria for lunch. Unfortunately, Victor Valley College did not have many places to eat on campus.

There would be a weekly market every Wednesday. The market would provide fresh fruits and vegetables, clothing, and a few Mexican food trucks. The trucks were famous for their spicy food and freshly cooked tamales. The cafeteria had an American restaurant that also included other cultural dishes. It was run by an Asian-American man who made it his family business and had a selection of Chinese food, Mexican food, and snacks for people on campus.

Many community colleges did not have the resources to house students, which brought a lot of incoming traffic to the cafeteria. If you were to come to the cafeteria at 12 PM, it most likely would be the peak of the restaurant rush, so it's probably best to go before 12 or after 1 PM. The staff at the college was tremendous, from the janitor to the president.

Even though everything did not go as planned, being at the college for almost a year and a half for Andrew, he enjoyed the opportunity and the experience he had. Walking around the city and being back was good and bad. Andrew felt as if he should have completed his program already. He should have been preparing at a division 1 program, working to become a great athlete for that upcoming season. But not everything in life is handed to you on a silver platter. Andrew soon realized how true that statement was and understood he had to keep working. The eligibility clock ticked and two and a half years of eligibility were left after graduation. He asked himself, should I keep going? Should I just graduate and say I am done with football? These were some questions that surrounded him in the first few weeks of the fall semester. Andrew kept to himself. The only people who knew about his offers and division 1 interest were only a few.

Being behind 9 months of expected graduation, there were only so many universities that wanted to invest their money into a questionable athlete. A questionable athlete is better known as someone who puts the program at risk either due to eligibility, illegal activities, or as simple as someone who has trouble following instructions. Andrew was a good kid, so he never was condemned for any misconduct, the only issue he had ever had since he finished high school was financial stability and eligibility.

Is an athlete only as good as the resources available to them? I can attest to this statement. If you do not have a great foundation, you are nothing. In current news, a building collapsed in Florida and killed hundreds of people sleeping. The individuals died because there was a lack of foundation. After all, the building engineers failed to build the proper stability before continuing to build.

Talking football, if you have ever watched a game, read about the sport, and most importantly, played on the field, you understand how important it is to have a great foundation. Andrew grew up poor, with no role model, and learned everything by himself and by observing. His path would have been more fluent if he had had resources for football camps and better guidance on his vision. The best offer in the fall was a small division 1 in North Carolina. The school was considered a small division 1 because it was in the FCS division; however, it was not a small school at all.

The university had over 13,000 students and was a powerhouse among HBCUs. The university was, in fact, the best HBCU in the country. A repeat MEAC and Celebration Bowl champion, the university shined a light on the universities in the area. He kept in contact with the offensive line coach and ensured to update him on his progress throughout the semester. It is amazing how you can go from over 20 division-1 schools interested in you to just 1. One thing to remember so far is the importance of eligibility and understanding what eligibility really is if you are a student-athlete.

The arrangements that were set up with Andrew got altered. There were ongoing issues of people taking care of the bills, and it was causing the need for relocation. Andrew's time was short; he only had 3 months left at the college. He knew he did not have time to waste; since he was not on the lease, he decided to leave the apartment. The situation was terrible to begin with; there were too many people in a small apartment, and the lack of maturity caused unnecessary problems financially.

A former teammate of Andrew that he played with in previous years, Adam, who lived on the second floor, the last apartment when you make a left after you get up the stairs in the apartment complex. When he went up there to hang out and catch up with a former teammate, he spoke to another roommate. The roommate he spoke to was a guy named Palo.

Palo was a young kid from the streets of Pasadena, California. Palo shared a room with his young two-year-old son Palo Jr., his child's mother Sara, and his girlfriend Denise occasionally. You could say he had a lot going on at the time. He was on the lease at the time and made most of the decisions for bills for the apartment. Andrew spoke to him and asked if he could sleep on the couch. He did not have much money; he only paid a few hundred dollars when he was downstairs in the complex and Andrew was homeless at the time sleeping in a tent near the college.

He agreed to 100$ a month and would need to give Palo the money on the 1st of each month. Andrew did not care about his surroundings; he just wanted a place to sleep while he tried to wrap up his degree. Andrew had all of his money tied to the college. He had roughly 600$ to last him 3 months. Andrew did not have anything at the time. He commuted by bus every day, blessed that it was free for students at the college. He used up 300$ to sleep on the couch, 200$ for food, and roughly 100$ left for anything else he may have needed. At this point, being homeless and hungry made him want to reach his goals sooner than later. If Palo did not offer him a place to sleep on the couch, there is no way he would have been financially stable to finish up his associate's degree and continue his bachelor's at a big-time university unless he wanted to come to class smelling like rotten eggs every day. Andrew probably would have done that just to finish what he started at least he was given a home for a few months. Who would pass up on 100$ rent for 3 months? The answer is no one. With everything good, there is always something bad.

The goal for Andrew as September was coming to an end, and he looked to his future was to graduate no matter what. If he needed to sleep in a sleeping bag, if he needed to sell his shoes, he would do whatever it takes. In his current situation, he had to deal with the environment right in front of him. Other than his former teammate Adam and the Palo family. The upstairs apartment housed 2 dogs, a Pitbull and a Chihuahua. There were 3 bedrooms, and on the first door, after you entered the apartment, there were 2 current football players: a linebacker and a defensive back. Those two young men were both freshmen in college. The last person who stayed in the apartment was a guy named Ajay.

Ajay was a sketchy character. He stood 5'5 and weighed 160 lbs., tatted all over his body. He had a long record of being in out of prison and also was a registered sex offender against a minor. He slept on a pullout mattress in the living room near the couch Andrew was on. In total, there were 10 people and 2 dogs, including Andrew, in a 3-bedroom apartment. The rent was cheap, so it sounded good until it did not. Everything began to change after a few days. There began to be a trend of miscommunication among the roommates. There was an ongoing issue between Palo and his child's mother. There were constant verbal arguments about responsibilities for their son. Palo felt as if Sara was not a good caregiver and was not doing what she needed to do to properly feed and shelter Palo Jr. when his dad was not there. The use of profanity and vulgar language was at an all-time high.

You could tell by his reactions that Palo had some anger issues. He punched walls, slammed doors, and had an excessive need to exert his voice when talking to females. It seemed as if he had some troubling wounds from his past and was overwhelmed throughout the day. Palo worked hard at a fast-food restaurant flipping burgers on most days of the week and was supposed to enroll in the following season's football program at the college with some of his other roommates. It got to the point where Palo became a cancer at home, constantly disturbing the other tenants with his loud outburst. If there was one thing that could be close to describing him was that he was a classic case of bipolar disorder.

His ability to go from a mild, calm, and collective voice and personality to an aggressive person who made it uncomfortable at times to be around him was extraordinary. He had a good heart, but he did not know how to express himself. Sometimes upbringing and how we were raised can determine our character and how we express ourselves. It was important to determine why we express ourselves a certain way; however, we should always have the ability to change it if it causes us to exude negativity. It got worse as the days passed by. Sara would constantly get beaten by Palo. It would get so bad he would drag her a couple meters from the bedroom to the front door and put her out of the home. Sarah sometimes would fight back, but he beat her like she molested someone in his family. He could not have ever loved the girl if this is how he treated her, especially knowing she was his child's mother.

She constantly told Palo, "I know I am nothing." You could tell her self-confidence was extremely low, and her outlook on life was at an extreme minimum. These were 2 people who dropped out of high school and were raised in corrupt low-income housing in California. Their surroundings allowed them to normalize violence when their surroundings should have normalized growth. Denise, who would show up occasionally, lived nearby. She would take the city bus until she reached the bus stop across from the convenience store. She would then commute down the street, passing crackheads and old men sexualizing her, and would proceed up the stairs to the second floor.

When she came in, the couple had a love and hate relationship. Sometimes they would stay up late when the roommates went to sleep and have sex, and sometimes they would have fist fights in the living room in front of everyone. Palo had no problem putting his hands on females; however, Denise was not like Sara, and she would constantly remind him of that. Denise would let Palo know she was not a punk and would punch him back. She refused to get beaten down and dragged out of the house like Sarah. The constant animosity caused roommates to feel there needed to be something done. The men in the house were tired of trying to calm down Palo and wanted a change to be made to make the apartment livable again.

Andrew was messed up mentally thinking about his future and thinking about his situation and was amazed at how he still was focused. More than anything, through all the distractions, Andrew remained focused. He tried his best to ignore the situations around him. Later on, as weeks went by, the guy in the living room was kicked out because he was sexually harassing some of the females in the house. It was funny how Palo was the center of this altercation; it did make sense since it was Sarah being harassed. The incident escalated between the two men, and Palo dragged him out of the house leaving Ajay with a cracked rib and a broken nose.

The previous day, Andrew had left early in the morning. He put on his headphones and continued his journey to the bus stop. Music was one of Andrew's go-to things. Being able to tune out the noise of the world and get into the rhythm of the music. Music was a way to meditate, and it could be therapy at times, depending on what situation he was going through. He had stayed late at the library that night, and when he left, it was one of the last buses leaving the college for the night. He did not mind being out all day. Getting out of the house filled with confrontation and bad energy had become a problem. He knew that if he was to leave the situation, he would be homeless. He could barely afford 300$ to pay for the rent. His decision caused him not to get involved in the altercations and to try to avoid the distraction by leaving early and coming back late.

The one time that Andrew felt bad was when Sarah sat beside him on the couch after she had gotten beat up by Palo, and Palo continued to proceed with the verbal outburst. She knew Andrew was big and could protect her if he wanted to, and she wanted to feel safe. Andrew regretted not protecting her because he knew he would be homeless if he had beaten up Palo. This was a lose-lose situation which you could only relate to if you were in Andrew's situation.

Andrew's fall semester was winding down, and he was getting on top of all his course material. He had emailed the coaches that were interested in taking a chance on him. Andrew had had San Diego State in the coaching office come in and speak with him. They were not showing much interest as they previously had because of his eligibility which was a pattern for the FBS level programs. He had become discouraged. He had some division 2 interest, but he knew he was much better than that. His confidence was still high because he knew his potential if he signed to a big-time school. Andrew had worked his ass off daily. He had 6 classes, worked out, and conditioned his body with everything he had.

"Opportunity waits on nobody" was his key self-talk quote. Believe it or not, it is what we live on. Do we believe we will be great providers and successful persons, or are we weak and do not aspire for a great future? Ask yourself this question and see how much it will tell you about yourself.

The only class that was giving Andrew trouble in graduating was geography. Geography class had been difficult because the teacher would talk fast and had an accent. Think back to a time when you had a teacher that may have been from a different country who spoke fast without the understanding that what was taught, the students heard something completely different. He was a lively man who created a fun dynamic in the classroom; however, he most definitely should have slowed down because there were other students with the same issue. Andrew had run into a little dilemma and was nervous that he would not be able to complete his class requirement. To achieve his associate's degree in psychology at the end of the fall semester, he needed to maintain a C in the class, and for some reason, he was having trouble passing the class. In his other courses, he had A's and B's, but in this class, he had a D.

The class was one of those courses weighted on attendance, exams, and a final project. These classes were good for college professors because it made it easier to grade large groups in a classroom. The only problem with courses being graded like this was that students did not have any room for mistakes. There was not a lot of material on which the grade was based, so he had to achieve an A or a B on every exam to complete the course and show satisfactory progress towards graduation. He had done terribly on the first 2 exams, but his attendance was excellent. He needed to get at least a B on the last exam and on the final project in order to finish with at least a C in the class. He spoke to the professor during office hours, and after they discussed what needed to be done, the professor gave Andrew an outline of the main topics for the last portion of the semester. Never be afraid to suck up your pride and ask for help; good people will always help you if you reach out. That is all that Andrew needed to get focused and engaged in preparing for his upcoming coursework. He was in a group of 3 and had to complete a PowerPoint presentation and outline: human influence on climate change. This topic needed sufficient research to be completed properly for his group to get a good grade. One group member was not into it and became a liability to the group. She avoided communication and would not attend group meetings; most importantly, she did not contribute any research to the final assignment. She, for some reason, was able to show up and come to the final presentation in front of the class. She did not want to practice, participate, or be involved; however, she still believed she deserved to get credit. Well, that is not how it works; for all the slackers who are lazy and like to piggyback off of someone's work that is not their own, go and look up the definition of research ethics and understand if you did not contribute to an assignment or a task at hand, you are not entitled to represent it as yours.

Back to Geography class, he was not letting it go down like that. Andrew knew how bad he needed to graduate; he also emphasized the importance of finishing this project promptly, which obviously did not get through to all of his group members. The lights turned off, the people in the class looked up to the monitor, and it was time for presentations. Next up was him. Andrew got up, and his other 2 group members joined. The one who was not involved in the presentation did not speak because, by the time the other group members spoke about the presentation, they made sure to leave nothing left for her. It was awkward since the professor asked why she did not speak, and Andrew told him what had happened. He was not about to give credit to a person with a terrible work ethic. One of his best characteristics was that he was self-driven and would do whatever it takes to reach his highest potential.

With only 3 weeks to graduate, it was decision time for Andrew. He had to create a plan of what to do with his future. It seemed as if he would just graduate junior college, and that would be the end of the road to his college football dreams. His division 1 football offers were gone, and he had no idea what to do. The one thing that made him think to himself, "this plan has to work," was when he flashed back to a few days before he left for college, and his absent father told him to not come back a disappointment. This statement allowed him to feel emotions, from anger to frustration to determination.

Determination was the key emotion he needed to get through that mental block and seek a positive outlook in the tough and challenging times. He prayed for a chance to impact and make a difference at a 4-year university. He was also motivated to continue because he knew that his mom had been in pain from the years of working so many hours each week. Blessed with an opportunity, he received a call from a great coach at a small division 1 school in North Carolina which had previously shown interest when all of his other division offers were non-existent. Coach Askins was a big 6'7 former NFL veteran who had played for several years in the NFL. He was a coach who had been a part of an HBCU dynasty in North Carolina. He had formerly coached an NFL pro tackle the previous year, and the program North Carolina A&T was ranked the #11 FCS football program in the country. This was the best opportunity at the time.

He was blessed to still have a division 1 offer and decided to capitalize on it; he probably should have waited a little longer. Right after he signed his LOI, he received an offer from the University of Tulsa, which was a jaw-dropping moment. He would have much rather capitalized on an FBS offer; it would have boosted his upside if he wanted to play pro football after he obtained his bachelor of arts in 2 years. He was thankful regardless and knew it was time to get right mentally and physically. He continued to train hard and work hard on finishing strong in the classroom. He graduated in December of 2018. He was able to move out of his apartment in Victorville, and he then left for Canada to be with his family.

It was a late Saturday night, and the flight left out of the airport and in Ontario, California. The flight was packed, and many people were traveling that night. Andrew sat in economy in an aisle seat. That was the best option for him if he was not in an emergency exit or first-class seating. The aisle seat provided extra leg room and created more mobility. It was still crammed; the service was mediocre, and he was ready to land. It seemed as if there had been a decrease in good service on some airlines. There were fewer good food options, and the planes were crammed and uncomfortable if you were a tall or big person.

Eventually, he landed in Toronto. It was wintertime, so the snow was falling, and a lot of mushy ice all over. Pearson airport was the main airport in the province. It catered to millions of people yearly and had accessible areas for disabled individuals with pick-up and drop-up services. Andrew got a shared ride; he did not want his mom to drive 20 minutes to pick him up when there was so much snow on the road. Another issue in Canada was that traffic could be backed up if the salt trucks did not come promptly during or after a snowfall. He put his luggage in the car and was on his way to Brampton to see his mom. He was excited. It had been almost 5 months since he left for California, and he needed to ensure everything was good.

Greeting him with a home-cooked meal was satisfying. He also left for a 10-minute drive to his aunt's house, who also lived in Brampton. She was there with his grandmother, uncle, and his little twin cousins. Everybody in that house was all over the place, they were in the bathroom, in the kitchen, and some were watching tv. He made sure to interact with everyone and spend a few hours before returning to his apartment and calling it a night. It was a long flight, and all Andrew wanted to do for the rest of the evening was get some sleep and wake up refreshed in the morning.

On a cold Wednesday night before New Year's Day, Andrew took a train from Brampton to London. The train ride was almost 3 hours and a snowstorm was taking place. The train moved so fast that you would have thought you were floating in the air. The trip was smooth. There were only a few travelers on the train that evening. People were sipping on their coffee, playing board games with their children, or watching movies on their laptops. Andrew laid back, had gotten some food before he traveled so he would not get hungry, and watched a couple comedy specials on his laptop. As the train pulled into the train station, he proceeded to get off the train. He then looked for a car that one of his good friends, Tom, was in. He came in a gray SUV with his little brother, and they waved to notify Andrew it was them. They proceeded to leave the station and went to Tom's house.

The music got louder as his little brother played his playlist on the car's Bluetooth. All 3 of them were having a good time, excited for the guys to be together for a few days. Tom's little brother's name was James. He was a 17-year-old senior in high school at the time. As they continued their ride down to the boy's parents' home, they were struck by a semi-truck on the right side of the vehicle. The car flipped over 8 times. There was glass, tires, and fire all around when the car came to a complete stop. The trucker had run a red light and was drinking.

The incident could have killed these 3 guys; with prayers, they survived their injuries. There were some stitches and some cuts and bruises, but nothing life-threatening. Long story short, the drunk driver was arrested and faced jail time. The boys recovered in a few weeks and were able to meet up again, but this time, it was to reflect on what had happened and go to the local gym for a workout and some conditioning and agility training. Tom played for a division 1 program, and James was looking to be a star at a university in Canada when he graduated. Everyone considered this a life lesson and continued to move forward with their training.

No matter what you go through, always have the mindset to move forward and do better. We only learn from our mistakes when we make them. A mistake is not a negative experience. It is a learning experience. Knowledge comes with wisdom. You can only become wise if you learn how to be knowledgeable. The key word is "learn." Be a person who can learn, and it is easy to transition into becoming a teacher when you have that open mindset. A teacher does not have to be a class instructor; a teacher can be a head of the house or any team leader.

In early February, there was an event that took place in an indoor dome. The dome had a large turf area and was a great place to host sports activities. Many young high school prospects attended the annual football showcase, which took place when everyone was together. Andrew and Tom spoke to the young boys and told them about their stories and how they overcame to have an opportunity to play division 1 football. It was a fascinating experience for the young men because they understood how their excellence level shined so much light and knowledge on these rising stars. It is important to understand that how you carry yourself can positively or negatively influence someone else. The showcase stars clapped after the men spoke, and it was their pleasure to watch them showcase their skills at the event later that hour. The men parted ways after the event. Tom and James drove back to London, and Andrew took a bus back to Brampton. Andrew stopped at the mall near his apartment when he arrived at the bus terminal. He grabbed some subway and was on his way home.

The goal for Andrew was to get to Division 1. Division 1 football hosted the best athletes in the country. Playing at that level gave a student-athlete the chance to get a shot to go pro. Understanding the importance of playing at that level, Andrew became more determined to continue battling his challenges. He was initially supposed to fly down to Greensboro, North Carolina, and practice with his team in February. If he did, he would have been able to attend spring camp and have time to learn the playbook before summer workouts.

On a quiet off day, after he had completed 60 hours during the week unloading boxes at a local warehouse, he sat alone in his room. In his room, he reflected on how many people were ahead of him, and he felt as if his value to an organization was diminishing. He found out from an email that was sent to him that the credits that he needed to be transferred were going through an evaluation process which was delayed. The processing time of this evaluation was extended by a few months.

Division 1 dreams were on pause, the spring semester start date had passed, and now Andrew and the coach had to decide what the best next step was. The decision was when it was done being evaluated, Andrew would get a ticket to come down to school. He could move into his apartment, get situated, and be medically checked out when he arrived. Still with high aspirations to continue playing football at a high level, Andrew trusted the process.

Sometimes in life, when it seems as if everything is detouring you from reaching your goal, that is when you have to have the willpower to overcome that challenge. For example, if you are defending your family in a fight, you can choose to flee, which does not solve the problem because then your family will not be secure; another option is fighting, fighting does not always mean you will win. With every loss, there is always a victory; victories do not have to be immediate but should be present at some point in time.

The hardest part for Andrew throughout these months was watching everyone move forward and still feeling stuck. The feeling of being alone and vulnerable was never present in his life, but at this time, this was what was right in front of him. He made the decision not to accept a scholarship in Canada. He chose not to settle for junior college or division 2 football when the road was getting tough. There is a song that quotes, "God gives his toughest battles to his toughest soldiers. Don't cry for me when the war is over." The meaning behind this statement is incredible. If you think deeply about this short sentence, you can understand a lot about yourself. Many of us are not fortunate enough to live a Hollywood lifestyle. Some of us cannot even afford a full gas tank.

The significance of God giving us tough battles is to see who will overcome them and give themselves the best chance of success and those who give up and allow adversity to steer them in the wrong direction. Working in a warehouse and taking the bus back and forth was becoming a norm that needed to break. Andrew was tired of struggling and tired of waiting for something good to happen. He did the best he could to be a good man, respectful and positive influence, and he knew something needed to happen, and it needed to happen now.

As the months passed by after his birthday, he received a notification from the local mail that there would be a package dropped off on the first Monday in May. When the day came, he went to the 1st floor of his 15-story building. He said hi to one of his neighbors in the building and opened the mailbox with his key. The mailbox usually had stuff he never wanted, like catalogs and coupons, which he disposed of, and behind was a letter from his transfer evaluation service. His excitement was throughout the roof.

He knew there was some news, whether it was good or bad, and he was looking forward to an update on his process. He pressed the button for the elevator: the apartment was only a few floors up. The elevator arrived, he hopped in and proceeded to his apartment. He began opening the letter and found the information he needed. He found out his transfer credits from his community college had been evaluated and were ready to be transferred and updated on his transcript. It was go-time now, he spoke to his positional coach and updated him on the process, and they worked on a date that would work.

After spring camp, a break took place; therefore, the best time for Andrew would be sometime in the summer. Andrew knew the earlier he could be at the university, the better. Andrew was a person who liked to be prepared regardless if it was in the classroom or elsewhere. The date was set for early July. Andrew thought the hard part was done but to no avail. He ran into some more issues. Andrew was now patiently waiting to leave in July. He was informed in mid-June he would need to sort out some additional paperwork before his student visa could be processed. The professionalism of the department at the university was not great when communicating with the potential student. A delay in responses and a lack of communication hindered the process. The process would take up to two months pushing his expected date back and making his arrival close to the 2019 season home opener. In late August, it was show-time. The process was mostly over, and now it was time to move forward, time to transition to something better.

# PART 3

–

# RISE AND FAME

It was Thursday morning, two and a half weeks away from the season opener against South Carolina State. Andrew left his apartment in Brampton, kissed his mom goodbye, and headed to the airport in Toronto. He got passed TSA and was headed down the escalator to his gate. The plane was boarding in 30 minutes, and he wanted to be on time. He sat down, looked in his backpack, made sure he did not lose anything and texted the team manager that he would be on his flight within the next hour.

The flight took off, and there were some drinks and pretzels offered on the flight. Andrew was not that hungry. He had eaten before he left his apartment. As he was in the air flying through Canada on his way to America, he sighed with a sense of relief. He thought the hard part was over, but his journey had just begun.

A couple of hours later, the plane arrived at a small airport in Greensboro, North Carolina. There were not many people at the airport nor on outgoing flights. The one thing that you can notice is that many people wore the Aggies' apparel.

'The Aggies' is a historical name from North Carolina A&T University. The name is not only familiar amongst locals but is well known in the south and east coast areas of the United States. The name's historical significance has been manifested since the nineteenth century. The university has been an institute of academic excellence and has carried a legacy of great athletes. Within the last few years, several athletes have been on an Olympic team, played on a professional roster, or achieved competitive salaries in their major.

Andrew was greeted at the airport by a short guy named Will. He was 4'11, had a strong build, and was excited to see the prospect safely make it to his city. They began their short commute to the university. They were able to familiarize themselves with each other and engage in what the schedule was for the upcoming weekend and fall camp. Will told Andrew that the offensive lineman was in the middle of a meeting from a long day of summer training, where he would be dropped off before doing anything else upon arrival on campus. Andrew could care less about meeting his teammates. The one thing he knew he wanted to accomplish that day was opening the Playbook.

The Playbook is like a freshly baked donut. A little bit crispy on the outside and soft and full of flavor on the inside. The Playbook has all that is needed to learn for most of the season. There still can be adjustments and added plays as the season progresses; however, the initial ideology of the team and the philosophy behind the games are within this book. When he finally arrived and hopped out, he saw a large stadium in front of him. He passed the locker room and athletic training office before heading to the offensive line meeting room.

As he opened his door in the meeting room, everyone was sitting in their seats, waiting for the coach to move on to the next play. The players heard about Andrews' arrival but thought it was a bluff. They were not expecting a junior college football athlete to arrive on campus right before the season started.

The men ultimately felt insecure and thought their job may be on the line. One lesson to take with you in life is that you may think everyone is on your team but pay attention closely, and you will see not everyone wants you to win. One aspect of today's society is there is a lot of jealousy and gossip. It might sound childish; however, take a second to think about it. Look at the news and research statistics on death in the last 10 years from jealousy. Many famous celebrities were killed because someone was jealous of their potential or success. In terms of gossip, what do people do at the largest universities, the biggest sports franchise, and the largest corporations?

The answer is they communicate. The real question is: are they effectively communicating or just looking for a way to defeat their opposition. I want to be specific to make sure everyone understands what I mean when I say opposition. Opponents can be a football team, company, or competing learning institution. Gossip can destroy an individual or a group because their energy is more focused on negative discussions about their counterparts, and they begin to lose a sense of themselves.

The best way to stay focused on jealousy and gossip is to shrink your group. Why do we need to have a big group of people as our circle of friends? The best answer is validation and seeking acceptance which most of us want. The people who do not seek validation and acceptance are the portion of the world we call leaders. Andrew was not a person to seek validation or acceptance. He was a leader in the way he spoke and in the way he carried himself; he ultimately despised followers and viewed them as cowards. Some of the teammates embraced him, and some did not. Not everyone is going to like you. It is as simple as that. Are you going to cry in the corner, or will you toughen up and say to yourself you do not care?

The truth is if a person is not making you money, feeding, and keeping your family secure, their opinion does not matter. Just because some people's opinion does not matter does not mean you should not consider their perspective. You just have to choose whose perspective you should give the time of day because it can be costly to you.

Andrew spoke up in front of the offensive line room and introduced himself, they ended the film session, and everyone walked out of the room. He spoke to the coach, got a big 100-page playbook, and headed to the parking lot. He was looking for one of his teammates to help him get situated; instead, it was his coach. For the first meal, they went to a local chicken spot, and then they went to the department store, and Andrew got what he needed for the semester and headed to the apartment with his coach. The apartment was on the lower of 2 levels. This apartment was fully furnished and had 3 bedrooms and 3 restrooms. There were no roommates in the apartment at the time; they arrived a week before the semester needed to begin.

Andrew finally got situated and removed all his belongings from the SUV. He began to look into his Playbook and tried to get a feel for the plays being run and the overall scheme of the offense. The Playbook was not easy to remember right away. There were many calls and different formations for different defenses that needed to be remembered. The cadence for the offensive line needed to be perfected; therefore, each lineman had to learn and practice with the QB through walkthroughs and practices.

The next day, Andrew proceeded with the football manager around campus. They needed to ensure he was properly situated with housing, health care, and a meal plan. The blessing was that everything was free because he was a full scholarship athlete. He had free books, free food, free rent, and free tuition.

There is always a cost with everything, and it was time for Andrew to learn nothing in life is free. If someone invests in you, whether as a business partner, a small investor, or free financial aid, there is always a need for a return on the investment. It can be anywhere from interest on a student loan to your individual contribution to a successful outcome. Andrew's contribution was how he played and performed at the university, determining if he would be valued at the program as an asset or considered a liability.

Division-1 programs all across America are preparing young men to be mature men. Maturity can be defined as being responsible for your actions. Maturity is to create a goal-oriented plan. Maturity is to understand that you are an investment and are only as valuable as your contribution.

The one thing that Andrew's coach said to him in a meeting during fall camp that he always remembered was, "We would love to have you, but we do not need you." As it would do to anyone, this statement did not sit well with him, it made him feel replaceable and not needed. He understood that at this level: it was a business, the highest level before pros, and the preparatory program available for college athletes was Division-1 football. Practice was violent. Every day, the boys were banging.

Toxic masculinity at its finest, a lot of trash-talking between players and coaches. A sufficient amount of profanity in one day to cover the entire country. Inside run, those 2 words you knew it was time to bang. Imagine fighting a grown man for position play after play, head-on collisions, and blood all over the place. Not many are able to be offensive linemen at the division-1 level; it takes tough, strong, resilient assholes to play that position. Every day you may have to deal with a defensive lineman complaining about holding when you have your balls in their face. You do not get any stats to show to your mom on posts on social media. If you are a real offensive lineman who at least started in high school, you can relate to the constant toughness needed to fulfill that responsibility.

When I say responsibility, I emphasize that along with any position on the football field. If you are on a scholarship or a contract, no matter if you are making not one dollar or 20 million dollars, if you are in that field, you need to respect the organization you are playing for and hold yourself accountable because no one else will. If you cannot do that, you will be replaced.

A replacement could be termination or reduction, and those two aspects are common in Division-1 football and professional football. You may get removed from the team or have funds reduced until you improve your value. One thing to remember if you are an upcoming high school player is you can and will be replaced if you are not contributing, there is no more cuddling, and that goes for anyone 18 or under. If you work or go to school, what happens if you do not perform at work or school?

The answer is you can be terminated from the company you are at, or they may require you to be retrained to meet standards. In terms of school, you can be on academic probation or kicked out of school. You are only valuable to society if you are an asset, not a liability. A good human does not want people that are liabilities around them, and no one wants to be liable.

Drill after drill, play after play, 1v1s, and team period: all came on a hot late summer day a week from the first game. Students began to get settled on campus, do dorm check-ins, and get situated with their registration. The campus vibe was beautiful; seeing the number of African American students was enlightening. If we know the history of HBCU schools, we could all have a profound respect for the development of each institution. The first HBCU was in Ohio and Pennsylvania before the civil war. The institutions were created because blacks were prevented from attending regular colleges and universities due to prejudice and racial discrimination. These institutions provided black youth opportunities to learn just like everyone else.

Everyone wants an opportunity. The only part that has been separating us is the concept of everyone wanting the person next to them to have an equal opportunity and not pass judgment on this simple concept that brings society together. African Americans could not get basic education, which helped begin the tremendous establishment of historically black colleges across the country. The only difference between HBCUs and regular universities when HBCUs came into existence was that blacks were not allowed to attend a regular college; however, an HBCU establishment has always been open to all races. It has never been right to prevent someone from reading and being literate. Why would you want to keep a race under you?

The answer is simple, competition creates intimidation. Many of us want to be alpha females and alpha males, but how can we achieve that when there is competition, most of us get anxious and nervous every time there is competition. It is understandable to have emotions, but it is time to approach competition as a challenge instead of something that needs to be shut down. When you approach competition as a learning experience, you are invested in finding ways to handle that competition in an effective way instead of a sudden quick response.

The battle of positions and getting ready for the season had begun. Many athletes had begun competing for a position as the travel roster was fast approaching. A level of competition and testosterone was at an all-time high. Everyone was trying to secure a roster spot and a position contributing to the team's success. Andrew had worked his ass off; he knew he had little time to learn the Playbook and try to compete for a position as an offensive tackle. There was a lot of hype around campus. Everyone was excited to have football back and the students back for the fall term. As the fall camp was ending and it was a few days from kickoff, Andrew was informed he would be a part of the active roster. He prepared for the season opener and was excited about his future.

The first game was here; it was a late 6-PM game at Truist stadium, and the crowd was ready. You could smell the southern BBQ from a mile away. A rich culture of pride was Aggies' land. Everyone in the community came out for the Saturday games. It was a place where people could feel safe, have a good time with each other and watch the football team take the field. The stadium was almost sold out, and it was the kickoff. The team ran out of the tunnel, the cheerleaders danced, and the drum line hit one of their classics, "I got 5 on it."

The stadium screamed in excitement, and now it was time to beat Elon and get ready for the big game of the year next week. The Aggies defeated the Phoenix in a close scoring shootout, 24-21, which was the end of week one. Like most Division-1 programs in the United States, Sunday was a rest day for the athletes, a time for treatment from the athletic trainer, and a way to meditate before the start of the week on Monday. The head coach spoke about focusing on 1 game at a time and the importance of staying consistent and building on previous mistakes.

The biggest lesson taught after week 1 is being accountable for yourself. Football is a team sport; however, there are 10 people, excluding the quarterback, who constantly have 1v1 matchups against the opposing offense or defense. The team trained harder, increased intensity, and mentally prepared for the challenge they faced on Saturday.

Duke Blue Devils, Wallace Wade Stadium in Durham, North Carolina's stage was set for the ACC showdown at 6 PM. The former HBCU FBS champions versus a rising FBS program that had just lost their quarterback in the draft, Jones was the 6th overall pick taken in the draft by New York. He played 4 seasons for the devils. Large buses boarded with the offense and defense. Before leaving campus, there was a ritual that happened to pay respect to the individuals who laid a foundation for historically black colleges. 4 men had been recreated into a statue. The statue was better known as February 1. This date and name came from the famous sit-in in 1960 of NCAT students who were getting lunch and faced discrimination. Their sit-in sparked outrage as there was social injustice. They inspired a future generation and influenced the progression of the struggle for civil rights.

Approaching the stadium, you would feel like you were in a movie if you were there. The biggest networks at the game, police escort with multiple cars surrounding the buses for the teams. Streets were empty and blocked off for miles. It was game time and time to see which men would be willing to fight the longest to get a win. As the gates were open, the Aggies entered the stadium. This was when the lights were the biggest. The huge stadium, which catered to tens of thousands of fans for years, was at full capacity. Everyone was seated, the stadium lights were on, and the referees had made it onto the field. Andrew and the boys got dressed up. They wanted to look really good. They had nice white uniforms and were ready to compete and show their worth. The boys came onto the field.

The leader of the team, Seth, had the boys ready for the competition. He shouted, "These boys ain't ready!" He repeated that statement as the men proceeded from the locker room, as he ran onto the field. No more talking; it was time for the coin toss.

The Aggies won the toss and decided to defer to the second half, which meant the defense was on. If you know football or have watched a defense come on after that team has won the toss, it is because they trust the defense, and it could be advantageous to receive the ball after the second half, especially if you do not have a lead in the game. The defense went lights out, dominating the Blue Devils. After that turnover, the Devils returned the favor. It was a close game in the first half, a back-and-forth shootout. The halftime performance was epic.

This was one of the university marching band's best performances ever. The Aggies shut down the stadium, and everyone was dancing, even the home team. The men came back on the field with the same energy. The offense wanted to start off fast and drive the ball down their throat, which they did in the first half. After the first drive, it seemed as if the defense went to sleep. The deep ball touchdowns were at an all-time high. The Aggies' cornerbacks could not lock up no one. The game was good overall, but after the loss, it was time for the Aggies to reset.

It is important after you fail, you do not get down on yourself but find a way to reset and try it again. A failure is only the amount of time you spend on it. A true professional player can overcome obstacles, small or large, because they have the mentality they cannot be broken, and their willpower will always support that argument. Back to the drawing board now.

It was Monday, week 3 of the season, and class began for the day. The students enjoyed the hot weather before the temperature dropped in a few weeks. Andrew was having some issues with the playbook; his coach was not as invested in his progression as he came close to the start of the season. As they added plays that were practiced throughout spring, Andrew had to memorize and be able to execute them in a matter of days. Andrew was also having trouble mentally. He was getting a little homesick, and his body was not used to so much banging daily. The term 'banging' relates to what happens for most interior lineman in football, they are constantly having head on collisions which cause wear and tear on their body especially at the division 1 level of college football. Andrew began going through a cycle, and it was not a good one. Andrew began to consume substances he should not to help him ease his stress every day. He also was using pain pills and alcohol to help with his recovery. He knew this was his last big opportunity, and he did whatever he could to be there with the boys on Saturday.

You could say he was showing signs of substance abuse which could lead to depression. He was struggling to learn the playbook, and some of the other players were able to advance to 1st team over him for the rest of the season. This caused

Andrew to go through a downward spiral. He was excited when he got on campus and was eager to be developed and reach his potential, but it seemed like this dream was meant for someone else.

This is the toughest thing to accept for some of us: the dream and goals we aspire to achieve sometimes are not meant for us. Nothing is wrong with having a plan b. Listen carefully. If you have a plan A and a plan B that can lead to success, there is nothing wrong with either option.

Andrew continued to work his tail off daily. He continued to grind out the season, getting himself back into the depth chart for playing on Saturday.

He eventually ended up winning two division 1 championships. He traveled to Atlanta, played in a professional stadium, and met many great people throughout his journey. As the semester was completed and the buses departed from Atlanta back to North Carolina, Andrew took a bus to the airport and flew back to Toronto to see his family for winter break. He was excited. It was a long time, and he needed a break from his atmosphere. There were a lot of family dinners and site seeing that took place over the few weeks. Andrew tried to create a game plan for the upcoming year. When he was done, he booked his one-way flight back to Greensboro, North Carolina.

As the spring semester was fast approaching, he made his visits around the city to see his family and close friends. The day was here, and it was time to return to school and settle for the semester. On the Tuesday before the Monday on which the term commenced, he flew out of Toronto in the afternoon. There was a lot of traffic, but there was no storm. That was a good thing because Andrew wanted to avoid any delays on his international flight. This semester, he had a full schedule. He was already situated in his apartment, and his meal plan carried over semesters. All he needed to do was show up to workouts and practice. The first month of February went well. Andrew was able to get into a good rhythm as the semester progressed. He was in the best shape of his life, and no one could have predicted what would happen next.

There were a lot of issues going on. There was a lot of discussion on campus about people getting sick, from the faculty to the athletes. Flu was being passed, something that rapidly could get to you and spread like wildfire. There was practice taking place for the football players, but Sheptism that the programs may be shut down to accommodate the virus. Andrew was going through his playbook on a warm spring day. He was getting ready for another two-a-day practice with his team. He began to research some type of sports enhancement that could benefit him on the field. HGH Somatropin is a way to help build muscle and lose body fat. He decided to try a cycle, and as soon as a shipment arrived the following week, he began to use daily injections. Andrews' mindset as he had a year of eligibility left, was that time waits on no one. He knew his father told him not to return a disappointment, his mother was always pushing him to play professional football. It was not discussed before, but Kesha made her son feel as if his only aspiration in life was him getting paid for football. She looked like she wanted a handout and wanted to get a return on her investment of having a son.

One thing to remember in life is you are a descendant of your parents, but your parents have the responsibility to let you find your way. This statement is so important in the wide spectrum of growth from teenagers to adulthood. Many parents want their children a certain way; instead, they push them away. This is not the parents' intention but the cause of their actions. As humans, once we reach 18, it is our choice and responsibility to be great contributors to society. We have the choice to overcome challenging situations, and we have the choice to surround ourselves with people who want to see us win.

The pressure that was given to Andrew made him think he was working on a short clock and he had to make an instant decision. Well, the enhancement did not serve much difference either due to incorrect treatment or the need for continuous cycles for the product.

It was pandemic time, and the amounts of deaths were increasing worldwide. Many students transitioned to online learning. Practices were being canceled nationwide for college athletes. Many faculty members had to take paid leave, and there was a need for some protection for the students. The facilities were closing down, and there was a late spring transition to online classrooms throughout North Carolina. Eligibility for Andrew and some of his teammates were pending. It was about to be a crazy road ahead for everyone. Schools were shut down, and football programs in America were stopped for the spring, summer, and fall 2020 semesters. The loss of pro coaches on campus was at an all-time high and everyone in the city of Greensboro was on lockdown or trying to stay safe with their family; therefore, it was the worst time to be scouted to play professional football. Seniors losing their last season, some people waited to hear if they could get their season of eligibility back. Some college athletes across the country decide to focus on their academics, graduate, and move forward in their life. The professional football combines, and pro days for athletes were canceled.

Athletes had to really focus on their plan B. Suppose you do not remember anything from reading this book. Remember to always have a plan B and make sure it is something you are passionate about for long-term fulfillment. What to do now? This was the question that Andrew faced. He had been almost out of playing football for over a year and a half. Was it time to move forward with his life or just continue chasing an empty dream? He had to make a choice and make it quickly. As the fall semester ended and most students across the country had transitioned to virtual learning, it was time for Christmas. This was one of the worst Christmases ever. The amount of rest in peace posts and family member interviews of lost loved ones were at an all-time high. This was probably the moment everyone knew not to ever mess with bats because the virus could have been caused because of the interactions with bats. Athletes across America were able to get a year back in eligibility if they had lost a year due to the virus. Andrew had spring coming up and had 2 options. Option 1: 1 summer and fall semester at a division 1 program or 2 full academic years at division 2. Now it was time for him to recruit himself again. He had not done so much recruiting since he left junior college 2 years ago. Faced with a decision, he probably emailed every football program at division 1 and 2 levels across the country.

Andrew's division 1 offers were gone. His eligibility was limited to one season at an FCS or an FBS program, and no coach in America wanted to take the risk of offering him a scholarship. What to do now? This was the question that Andrew needed to figure out. Andrew still had 2 years of eligibility left at a division 2 program, and he needed to finish his degree at the minimum. Andrew did not want to come all the way to the United States, go through the process, and not have anything to show for it. He had committed to Western Colorado University as it was his last academic year as an undergraduate student. He had planned to go over to Colorado and get acquainted sometime in August and play a complete football season. This was Andrew's first time back in college since the pandemic. It had been an exciting time for him. Andrew had been excited to leave the house and be on the go again. He had felt lethargic being in lockdown a state over and needed to feel a part of something again. Andrew had been excited to earn his bachelor's degree in psychology. He could bring home a degree he valued more than playing professional football.

Many athletes focus on going to college with the aspiration of going pro. When athletes should be using sports to get financial aid to support college, college needs to be the goal, and graduation needs to be the result. After you graduate college, you can do whatever you like. You can play professional sports if you are a part of the 1%, go into a career, or use that experience to help you further your education. The point is that upcoming athletes should not go to college to play professional sports; instead, they should use athletics to fund their education.

August had come around, and it was time to see what Western had. Western Colorado University was located in Gunnison, Colorado, 3 hours from Denver, the home of many professional teams. Gunnison was in the heart of some of the world's most beautiful mountains and landscapes. Gunnison, Colorado, had less than 7000 people and almost 8000 ft in elevation, making it one of the highest elevated cities. The breathing conditions make it almost unbearable for out-of-state students who are used to sea level air quality. The air quality is thick and can take a period to adjust. Many students at the university enjoy skiing throughout the year and visiting national parks nearby. The school caters to many Gunnison locals who want to be a part of the field house. The field house allows members to do aerobic training, 1-on-1 workout, and rock climbing. The city is predominantly Caucasian, with only a few hundred people from other ethnic backgrounds. One thing that many people may not be prepared for is the extremely cold weather over the winter months. Gunnison is known as one of the coldest cities and one of the most beautiful places in the country.

Andrew was to have reported to the school a week before summer camp. He had the entire summer to train and get back in shape for his last year of football and also his last academic year, which he intended to graduate in the spring. He drove from Las Vegas to Gunnison with one of his teammates, a freshman offensive lineman whose name was Pete. They commuted 10 hours late at night and arrived early in the morning. They went to the local store and got some stuff for Andrew's apartment and his teammate Pete. Pete was also a barber, so he gave him a haircut. The following day it was time to get more acquainted with the coaching staff and try to get acquainted with some of the players who arrived back on campus for camp in a few days.

Andrew began conditioning and stretching. He was trying to get adjusted to the hard-to-breathe elevation. The elevation was no joke, one of the most difficult places to breathe and play. Remember, Andrew, at this point in his life, had played all over Canada, Texas, Florida, North Carolina, and California; however, Gunnison was the most difficult because it required you to be in impeccable conditioning.

On Saturday, when it was time for the conditioning test, Andrew did not make the time needed. He could barely breathe; the ridiculous part of him failing is that he timed himself completing the test at a lower elevated state and completed it. The question is: is it good for athletes to play sports in a highly elevated city? The answer is no. The amount of conditioning and water intake needed to be stable and not pass out is remarkable. You can drink 2 gallons of water and still be dehydrated. That might have been an exaggeration, but is it really? You need to run and exercise in such circumstances to understand and be able to relate to what is being discussed. Andrew had to go to the hospital at the beginning of a camp to get an inhaler prescribed because he was having trouble adjusting.

The camp days went well. Andrew learned the playbook and competed for a position with the mountaineers. The season progressed, and it went well. The team was pretty good, and they went 10-1. Andrew got some good film and was able to win a championship and celebrate with his teammates. The team spirit was tremendous. It was a diverse team: for the most part, there were Caucasians, African Americans, and some Latino players. The team had great chemistry on the football field and off. The players genuinely cared about each other; they would shut down Gunnison every Saturday with some of the most epic parties ever. The people at Western most definitely knew how to have a good time. The cohesiveness was why the football players won a championship in November 2021. The crazy thing about this semester was that Andrew was a part of the football team, but he was dealing with a lot at the time. One of his mentors passed away and it had been pushing for 3 years since he had seen his family.

Every day, Andrew would walk an hour to the school from his apartment; sunshine or snow, it did not matter. After practice, after games, and 2 am after a road game win, he had no other option. Some days he may be able to get a ride, but he had too much pride to ask for handouts. Andrew would, at times, walk with his book bag, a gallon of water, and 4 bags of groceries and walk 30 minutes in -20 weather. It did not matter. He was committed to the program and knew he only had 2 semesters to get things done and get his life in order. Every day he would walk on campus like everything was great; he tried to make everyone feel included and invited. He would start conversations with everyone in the class and always make them laugh when he hurt inside. Andrew never had a good father figure. He had professional dreams that went left after the pandemic, and his support system was not in existence; it did not matter. In spring 2022, he needed to graduate, and that was the only goal. If you focused on a goal because it is all you had to attain, distractions did not matter.

There were a lot of locals that would look at him walking around like he was not supposed to be there. He would get stares from people when he walked into a grocery store or anywhere. The way people looked at him in this city was as if he did not belong. He was called an outsider by a lady in Gunnison, and some of the people in the city would speak to him like he was a second-class citizen; it could have been because he made up 1% of the minorities, who were either Latin or African Americans, or because he was 6'4 and had tattoos. However, Andrew's response would be him putting his headphones on and going on with his business. Andrew woke up at 5 am throughout the regular season, got ready, and headed to the team workout. He balanced 6 classes in the fall and would have to balance another 6 classes in the spring to graduate at the end of the academic year. It was getting more challenging as the semester continued. Eventually, he could get to finals and complete his requirements for that semester. With every tough battle, there is always a way to overcome that difficulty. He took the challenge and really never gave up.

During the winter break, Andrew drove with one of his friends, Amanda, who was African American. She was in California at the time. He went through a middle-class neighborhood. It was diverse, so he felt safe and was not worried about any odd encounters. Sarah worked for a delivery company and would pick up food ordered online and be responsible for getting it to a customer. Andrew was driving, and Amanda was in the passenger seat with the customer's meal. They pulled into a large gated community and entered the code provided. The gate opened, and they proceeded through. On their way to the customer's home, you could see that the neighborhood was fairly quiet. It was a little after lunch on a weekday; therefore, most of the homeowners were probably out or at work.

Amanda left the black Honda and went to the door, and placed it on the step. She then proceeded to take a picture and head back to the vehicle. Amanda shut the door, and the two friends were off to the gate to get out of the property. A white SUV with two Caucasian females pulled their vehicle in front of Andrew and Amanda, blocking their view of the gate and blocking the main intersection for the gated community. The women were on the phone calling the police. They told them there was a suspicious vehicle and that they were not a part of the neighborhood. Andrew and Amanda begged them and pleaded to them they were there dropping food and had no intention of doing anything to their community. They did not care. All the females saw was a pair of African American friends with a black car somewhere they did not live in.

The police arrived quicker than ever. They took Amanda and body slammed her on the ground. They broke Andrew's phone and tased him for not complying. Without evidence, the officers were able to put them in 2 separate cars for questioning. By the grace of God, the Caucasian family to whom the food was delivered were able to talk to the officers allowing the friends to be released with only a simple apology. Without any money for a lawyer or legal representation, the friends were not able to have the incident investigated further.

Money. Money. Money. The world revolves around money. It is all about who you are and what you can contribute. The sooner an individual can understand this concept, the better off they will be. You can try to attract people with your personality but what they really want is your financial resources. Start saving at least 20$ a month in a savings account as soon as possible. Get your money up if you want to be free from discrimination and judgment. People respect success, and when you have credentials or important people supporting you, you simply do not have to deal with prejudice as often if you are poor and if you lack resources.

After New Year's Eve, it was time to start getting prepared to head back to Colorado for the beginning of the spring semester. Andrew decided to drive back with one of his teammates, who stayed out in California the day before the semester started. The commute took 15 hours. Back on campus, Andrew was ecstatic about the new semester and the last semester of his college experience in the United States.

Andrew was taking 6 classes and 2 online at the time. He was engaged in his commitment to finishing off strong and looking forward to his future. He still had one more year of eligibility to play football; however, he was getting interest from Canadian professional football teams to play back at home. He decided he would continue working towards graduation and see where the chips land. It's crazy how people can be so dismissive of racism and encourage laughter towards a culture to normalize prejudice. Spoken by some college professors and teammates was the former president's dismissal. Here is the story: the president walked into a room where students were and stated, "It is too black in here," the president came to a mutual resignation.

He still got paid millions of dollars, he had free housing, and they wrote a false news article claiming he had got dismissed for something else to cover up his incompetence as a leader. The way the university staff discussed the details about the incident of the former president with such little regard for how ignorance and racism can affect the people around them diminishes the integrity of people's values. The university is not to blame for people's thoughts. Many universities deal with sexual assaults, misconduct in research, and racism against students. The change of perspective starts with education. Education of cultures enhancing the love for diversity is what educational curriculums have missed for centuries. Why not have a class on diversity and equality in the world and workplace in every high school and undergraduate program. There should be a requirement to take this class at least once in the 4 years of high school and then once in the 4 years of university.

What's crazy was that there was a student named Jeremy who had a class with Andrew. He was on the soccer team, and he was a good guy. He had great value in his motor development class discussions in the fall. He was an African American athlete who was from out of state. He was one of the few African American students at the university. A notification that was sent to students indicated Jeremy jumped off a bridge nearby and fell 80 ft to his death.

His family, who spoke to some of his teammates, emphasized he was going through a lot being a black athlete at a predominantly white institution. Jeremy was always positive, but he struggled to fit in. Sometimes he would pass people in the community and get racial remarks towards him.

Jeremy wrote a note saying to his family, "I love you. God gave me a chance, and I know this is not what you want. But I can't do this anymore." The funeral arrangement happened a few days later, and people who knew him showed support; everyone else he knew seemed to have moved forward in their lives.

People only value you as your contributions to them and to their cause right now. We can look at famous athletes who have died, and we see how quickly we forget their contribution. It is important to stay present at the moment. Allow yourself to have short-term and long-term goals; however, you need to focus on now and what you can achieve right now.

Looking towards the future, Andrew was 2 months from graduation. The commitment he showed to doing whatever it took was remarkable. His resourcefulness, confidence, and leadership showed he was ready for anything life had in store. Throughout his few semesters at the university, he stayed in a 2-bedroom apartment. The apartment was near a farm where an old man lived and would also take care of his animals. He would wake up early in the morning and let his horses out and make sure the grass was cut to perfection. In Andrew's apartment, he stayed with an older man named James.

He was not old; he was just older than Andrew. He was a 27-year-old freshman. Nothing is wrong with going to college at any age. Just know how to act your age. James would not go to class, he slept with bed bugs, and he had hair lice. He would not shower for a week at times and still attend the university. His stench would travel all over the house. James was just a delinquent. It is as simple as that. Without any home training, he was a distraction to Andrew.

The lesson he learned in this situation is to keep moving forward because no one cares. In life, we face distractions and people who are not on the same path as us. As a man or woman, you must stay committed to what benefits you and remove yourself from what does not.

Creating expectations was what came next for Andrew, expectations in the classroom, his career, as well as physical and mental health expectations.

Train your body as much as you train your mind. Wake up in the morning and do 30 minutes of cardio and 30 minutes of strength training for 3 days weekly. Eat a portion size less than usual daily for a year. Drink a gallon of water every day. Work on the small changes and watch your long-term goals become short-term.

Do you remember the question – discussed at the beginning of the book – is it possible for a student who had a 1.9 GPA after high school and lost many opportunities to achieve a 3.75 GPA and graduate on the Dean's List?

Well, the answer is: Yes, it is possible. Through patience and hard work, Andrew graduated with a 3.75 and achieved a 3.8 in his last term, receiving his bachelor of arts degree in psychology, achieving institutional honors Magna Cum Laude.

# A LESSON TO BE LEARNED

Everyone wants to be at their best, which means at their peak. The top is only for a few, but why? Why can't everyone get a piece of the pie? Why do we, as people, alter our values to fit in? Why are we capable of displaying hate as much as we show love? Why do we abuse each other and expect to be rewarded? Why are we surrounded with jealousy when we were created at birth equally? Ask yourself these questions and see what you come up with.

Andrew started off with nothing. No consistent father figure, living in poverty, and gun violence. He was able to get reformed at a private school and begin playing football with his friends when he moved cities. He stuck to the road with whatever distractions were in his way and kept going. Andrew won 3 college championships, became one of the best offensive linemen when he was in college, and lived his dream of playing division-1 football. Andrew lost it all and gained success in his education as a plan B. If this is not a story of keep moving forward and not give up, then what is?

Keep grinding because your time is coming, and either you will be ready for that moment or you will not; therefore, make a choice not to quit and give in to mediocrity.

# 5 FIGHT-OR-FLIGHT RESPONSE EXERCISES

1. If you are in a confrontation and you have loved ones near you, leave the situation. Their safety is more important than yours.

2. In a heated moment in your life, breathe in and out and do it 5 times. Keep doing it every time you face a heated moment. Make it a routine and a resolution to calming your thinking.

3. If you are in a tough environment, it could be poor or competitive, focus on the process and keep moving forward. Do not run away from a challenge.

4. We all want success but are we willing to do what needs to be done? Ask yourself this when you create an idea or if you want to achieve something substantial. You can choose to fight and overcome or leave when it gets hard; therefore, make that choice.

5. If you feel like you lost everything or are on track to lose everything, you can say, "I am done, and I have accepted mediocrity," or you can grow some backbone and speak that fancy house dream into reality. As I will continue to emphasize, we all have choices. Make the right one.

# ACTIVITY PLAN

A 16-week plan for students in high school, undergraduate, and graduate programs with 48 classroom exercises and activities. The activity plan can also be used for team-building exercises anywhere there are 6 or more people.

Complete 3 activities per week for 16 weeks to get the best results. You do not have to be a student; you just have to have an open mind. Great for group therapy sessions. Participation is recommended for anyone over the age of 12. Instructors should prepare activity plans 24 hours before.

## Challenges

1. Discussing past and present challenges and how the future outcome needs to be influenced for peak performance.

## Trust Fall

2. Trust fall exercise with someone that looks the least like you or someone you do not know.

## Presentation

3. 2 groups. Stand on 1 leg for 1 minute. The losing group has 5 minutes to come up with a verbal presentation about a topic relevant to the course.

## Understanding The Material

4. Circle up in a large group or separate the class into 2 groups. In this activity, there will be one representative from each group or 2 for the entire class. The discussion will be about effective strategies for using the course material toward a career. The discussion should be no more than 10-15 minutes.

## Set A Timer

5. Everyone in the class needs to close their eyes. Set a timer for 2 minutes. Look at what the 'students' body language is. If a student is engaged to participate, put them in section A of the classroom, which would represent a positive section. If they seem not engaged and are waiting for the exercise to be over with, put them in section B of the classroom, which will be negative. The objective is to ask section B how much do they care about the course they are in on a scale of 1-10? If anyone in this section records a 5 or under, there is a good chance they are not engaged in the material being taught. This can be anonymous and written on paper. Ask section A why is it important to care about the course they are in? This can also be anonymous and written on paper. This is a simple but effective way for teachers and professors in the first weeks of class to better understand their students' commitment in the classroom without them knowing it.

## Conquering An Obstacle

6. The exercise will require strategy and will be useful for team building. The students should all be working together for a common goal. The students can also go outside if they need to. The class should have a few desks or chairs, and they should be beside each other. The spacing between the chairs should be large enough for the entire body of students to stay in front of the chairs. There should be an imaginary line that is roughly 1-2 feet in height. Having access to duct tape or a thick string will make the game more fun. Attach the tape or string from the start of chair 1 to chair 2. The objective of the exercise is for the students to be aware that the chairs and line which prevents them from crossing is an obstacle they need to overcome. We can imagine the line will shock them if they touch it. Make sure everyone who participates holds hands. Closes their eyes and crosses. Have one or two people guide the class. This team exercise is good for bringing cohesiveness to the classroom.

## The Large Twist

7. This is a fun game that creates unity and allows your class to bond for the common good of an activity. Students should stand in a circle holding hands with each other. The goal of this exercise is for students to walk everywhere; it can be above, under, or in between each other. Create a knot. The objective is to untangle that knot while keeping everyone still holding each other's hands. This exercise is great for communication in the classroom.

## Escape Room

8. Create an escape room in the classroom. Let the students find different items in a class you have set up for the common goal. The goal is to puzzle everything together to be able to leave the classroom. You can make this into a competitive class setting by dividing the students into two groups. This is a fun activity that will bring the best out of your students and show which students are leaders and which are followers. As a teacher, it is important to develop 'students' learning experiences by creating leaders. After the exercise is completed, ensure you work on cnhancing the skills of the weaker students in each group.

## Stepping Stones Of Yourself

9. In today's society, there are different levels of success. If a person wants to grow and think positively, they must be molded and motivated to be that person. Creating and planning are essential ways to achieve and keep achieving success, which is normally the objective for many. In this exercise, the students will be divided into 4 groups. Use either toothpicks and marshmallows, or if you have a set of Lego pieces, that can work as well. Let the students work together to build a structure. The best one wins. It does not have to reach a certain height; it just has to have the most detail. This activity is great for students to focus on every specific attribute of the structure. This skill is important if you want to be stable in any position in life. If you pay attention to the fine print and emphasize the details, you will always have a more precise outcome.

## Tell Me Something Creative

10. Students should be in a circle for this activity. It is important to enhance students' creative thinking. Start with something simple such as a place or city. The instructor should start the narration and allow a student to continue where the story left off. Every student should be able to participate and contribute to the creative process of the timeline for the story. At the end of the story, it should be something special that you and the students have worked on together. An instructor can relate it to a relevant topic in class if they would like.

## The Walls Are Caving In

11. In this game, the walls are caving in. The classroom should be divided into two groups. The instructor needs to create a small space that each group must all fit in. There should be multiple spaces as each group advances. The objective for the group is how many people can fit in the smallest space wins. An example is using a rope or duct tape to create a barrier for students to get into. Making the best out of a bad situation is the lesson for the students to learn from this activity.

## Organization

12. The students must decide which way to organize themselves. Some good recommendations are by height (low to high), feet size (low to high), or weight (low to high). They only have 60 seconds and one chance to do this activity. If they make it before the 60 seconds, they win that round. The objective is to see if the students can communicate effectively in a short time frame. Run the trial again with a different factor. This exercise aims to allow students to think suddenly and develop their quick thinking and response skills.

## It's Time To Celebrate

13. This is good exercise around a holiday or a day off of class work. Prepare this activity at least 24 hours in advance. Let the student know you want them to bring at least one item to celebrate with their class. It could be something simple as a 2-liter soda, a deck of cards, or a bag of chips. Everyone must participate. The entire classroom loses the reward if someone does not bring an item. It could be a reward such as 10 extra points towards a grade which should be announced before the students buy or bring their item. If a student who does not agree to bring an item still brings an item to the classroom, the student does not lose the competition for his or her class; however, if one person who agreed to bring an item does not bring something entirely, everyone loses the reward. The goal of this activity, as you probably predicted, is accountability. One of the biggest words, not the most difficult, is accountability. Accountability comes from being aware that you have a responsibility and that you should execute it as required. This can be at your job, as a head of household, or anywhere you are valued as an asset. This can be a fun exercise and rewarding exercise, but it may not end in a reward. It depends on the accountability of each student.

## Flip A Coin

14. Divide the class into pairs. Give each pair a coin. Let them flip it 5 times each after they guess what it is. If they achieve more than 80% or ⅘ of what they flipped correctly, put them in the category of luck. The others who had less correct put them in the category of hard work. Most likely, the luck category will only have a few students if done correctly. The goal of this exercise is for students to understand that only a few of us can be lucky in today's growing society. Most of us will fall under the category of having to work hard to reach the same status as those who live based on luck. This exercise is proven because the group of students that are in the lucky category if you were to test the experiment again, you would see the difficulty of achieving 80% of the coin flips in a re-trial.

## Let's Make A Film

15. Create a class movie. For this exercise, students must create a plot for a film relevant to a topic discussed in class. Once the clock starts, each student will have 3 minutes to create a scene for the movie. It should be, on average, 3-5 sentences. After the time is up, the students must piece together the scenes into one big movie. The goal is to have the best movie script possible with a good flow to it. Give them 10 minutes and set a timer. This exercise aims to let students think creatively and critically for a bigger picture.

## Obstacle

16. Divide the class into 2 groups. Each group will be required to use 5 pencils or pens, a string, and a roll of tape. Each group will have 8 minutes to create a free-standing object. The objective is to see which free-standing object is the tallest with the use of strategic strategy amongst the class. This exercise is great for team building which is essential for projects and positive class interactions.

## Create A Maze

17. Use objects in the classroom and put them on the floor in a pattern that starts and leads to the exit. There will be pairs of students for this exercise. One blindfolded and one that will be an instructor. The instructing student must guide the blindfolded student to the exit in 60 seconds before the lion comes and eats the student. The pair with the quickest time wins. The goal of this exercise is to be able to communicate when it is not the best situation. The benefit of this type of communication is for people who are athletes or plan on going into careers that are under tremendous pressure to communicate effectively to bring the best outcome of a challenging situation, such as the military or being an active-duty officer.

## Social Skills

18. Trade your pencil and pen with someone else for the day and require everyone to be comfortable sitting in a specific seat throughout a lecture that is different from their normal seating. When the student moves and trades utensils, they should not just simply sit down and not verbally engage. Each student must ask the new person their name, their career goal, and what is the benefit of diversity and effective thinking?

## Speak Up

19. In corporate and similar industries, it is all about relationships; therefore, engaging in a classroom and getting your students' attention is extremely important. Being relatable and respectful is what can help a mediocre student become an overachiever. A great activity is asking students to stand up and speak about one thing they can't live without and one person they cannot live without. The teacher should also engage in this discussion. After everyone answers, there should be a projected screen, or you can write and illustrate on the classroom board why we feel we need to live on earth with certain people and things. The objective is to get to the necessary needs we all want as humans. For example, safety, belongings, and social support. After this exercise is done. Ask the students whether or not there is a difference between wants and needs? Then follow up by discussing the many things we may want that are not needed. The people that we may want around us and the material things do not always lead to success. It is important to have the people you need in life. This statement is important to encourage students who plan on pursuing a demanding career in relationships, whether an employee and boss or a wife and husband. We may want a certain connection, but it is not needed if it does not serve the sole purpose of having a successful outcome.

## Z-Pattern

20. Get some cups. It is recommended you prepare for this activity beforehand. Each student should be divided into pairs. You will need at least 10 cups in the shape of a *Z* with spacing in between. 1 blindfolded or with their eyes closed, and the other student should be the instructor for this exercise. The visually impaired student should have limited space to work with and must go either over the cups or around them. They should not be able to hit other students near them trying to avoid the cups. You can put duct tape lines that will serve as barriers for the Z-shaped cup pattern. The objective is to be the fastest pair to the finish without hitting any cups. If you hit a cup, you start over. That means each person in a pair should participate. There should be 2 races and a timer for each. The goal is to allow students to think quickly and effectively while working together. In every great company, the most effective and productive is the team that is quick and has great communication.

## Eye Contact

21. Get the students into pairs. Let them stare at each other in the eyes without blinking. The person who lasts the longest wins. The students who win should be paired again with someone else who wins. Keep going as a process of elimination. The last person standing will be the champion of this exercise. The goal of this exercise is for students to be comfortable with being uncomfortable. Students need to be able to have eye contact while communicating with adults. It shows confidence and demands respect.

## Illustrate Your Best Idea

22. For this exercise, students must be divided into groups of 3. The instructor will give 1 out of 3 members in the group a picture of a person to illustrate discreteness from the rest of the class. A family member is a recommended option for instructors. The person, after being instructed, will sit down and draw that picture. There will be 1 out of 3 group members who should not know what is being drawn or what is supposed to be drawn. You can put the ⅓ of the classroom somewhere else. The last ⅓ of the classroom will be responsible for watching over the person drawing. The first picture will take 3 minutes to draw. After the time is up. The person watching the drawer must relate the information based on how the picture looks without identifying who that person is to the student who was a part of the ⅓ in the classroom who does not know anything going on. That person will have 4 minutes to come up with the exact drawing of the initial image. There should also be no communication with the first drawer once the student has completed their 3 minutes. The class can judge the best pairs of pictures at the end of the 4 minutes. Most similar pair of photos in each group of 3 wins.

## Identifying Cognitive Distortions Then Restructuring Them

23. For this activity, the student is responsible for shifting their thinking at a sudden response. This is a fun exercise that may get loud, so be aware. Cut the students in half. Let them find a partner or assign them one. The pairs will be given 60 seconds each to say as many pairs of words as possible. The pair of words will consist of: 1 negative thought, each student's partner must say the opposite of that word, which would be a positive thought. For example, failure (negative) versus success (positive). The pair of students with the most words in 60 seconds wins. Positive reinforcement is always good. Therefore, make sure that the winning pair has some type of reward. This is a powerful exercise to allow students to think positively when they are surrounded by negative thoughts.

## What Are You Thinking About

24. A record of each student's thoughts is important for developing their thinking and how they process problems. This exercise is useful for developing a person's problem-solving quickness and resourcefulness. The exercise will consist of 10 bad thoughts and 10 that are good. Their thoughts should all be about what has happened in the last 48 hours. The next step will be for students to say I will let go of negative thoughts and do what I have to, to be successful. They will repeat it 3 times after they complete their thought record.

## The Thinking Tree

25. The thinking tree has been strategically formulated to help students change their thoughts. The goal is to change the thoughts that may cause sadness or negative emotions. Each student must draw a tree with 10 branches on a piece of paper. They will rank their deepest concerns, starting from #10 and ending at #1, with 10 being their biggest concern. Each student will only have 90 seconds to complete this task. As the students begin working on the exercise, you will see that they will have trouble creating this tree as it is hard to have 10 overwhelming issues and think of it in a short amount of time. After the exercise, a student may get a different perspective. After the student is done, tell them to write down 1 effective strategy that can ease stress in a challenging or overwhelming situation.

## Create A Story

26. The class will be divided into two groups, and the responsibilities of those groups are to create a story related to the course they are in. Each group should pick a relevant topic and show a timeline from the beginning until the end. For example, this story can be an outline of an experiment or a business plan. The students should be able to demonstrate how the completed assignment is relevant to a topic discussed in class.

## What's Next

27. Each student has 10 minutes to list 10 careers that can come from their course and write a short 1-sentence description of each career. This class exercise is useful at the beginning of a class. Even if the student does not plan on going to a work-related field in that specific career, they should not go through the entire class without understanding the benefits of learning the course material, which will be understood more when the students can relate it to specific careers.

## Create A Plan

28. Make a plan. This is an important part of any learning objective or aspiration for long-term success. Understanding how to plan out your life effectively can create a stress-free environment and develop great habits that will help you in a respectable career. Each student should spend 20 minutes working on a plan for this exercise. The plan can be anonymous and handed in at the end of the class or submitted online. The plan should have 3 main sections: short-term goals, long-term goals, and effective strategies for achieving them. The plan should be at least a page long written.

## Breaking Down Barriers

29. Why are there different levels in society? This is a discussion that is controversial but needed.

    In 2022, we face many disagreements and different views as a nation. It is important to understand why there are different levels in society. Divide the class into two groups and label one group as the low class and the other as the high class. The objective is for each group to prove why their given class is needed in society. This exercise aims to get students to understand that it is important to respect everyone because everyone has a responsibility and value. To better understand this concept, conceptualize a garbage driver quitting his job or the CEO of an important water supply company resigning. If they are not available, both individuals can cause a problem in the flow of society, creating a shortage and need for additional resources. Make sure the students understand the importance of both classes.

## Ask Some Questions

30. Pop quiz time. Ask the students 10 questions related to content throughout the semester. At the end of the pop quiz, ask the bonus question: name one exercise or activity discussed throughout the semester that was the most engaging and useful?

## Relax Your Mind

31. A meditation exercise will be a great way to start the class and create a relaxed dynamic among the students in class. In the first 5 minutes of the class, ask everyone to take a deep breath in and out. Then ask them to close their eyes for 60 seconds. When everyone has finished, tell them to say one word about how they feel. The objective of this exercise is to get your students mentally ready for classroom discussion. This exercise may be useful at the beginning of a quiz or exam.

32. Never be afraid to ask tough questions. Divide the class into groups and ask one side to come up with reasons why it is important to work well with others in a group session? Ask the other side of the room why people have difficulty working well together? The objective of this task is to come up with effective ways of working with others. This exercise is one of the most important in this book. Not only does a typical person need to be able to work well with others they, at times, have to depend on others throughout life. Working well with others, regardless of ethnicity or economic status, can separate a mediocre achiever from a successful figure in today's developing society.

## Resume Building

33. How to make an effective cover level and resume. This is an essential skill that should be taught in every class. Let each student have 20-30 minutes in class to complete an outline of a cover letter and resume. The objective is to have the subheadings and the correct formatting and be able to get their credentials together to complete this task. You, as an instructor, should be able to follow a common format that everyone can lead with. Even if the curriculum does not require this skill, giving your students the foundation can be crucial to their development in academic and career success.

## Building Connections

34. 10 professionals are the concept for this exercise. Each student should be able to come up with a list of 10 professionals in the career of their choice in the city or state they are in. The students should only use the professionals if they have credibility and have a way of contacting them. The objective of this exercise is to get students to network. The goal of the task is for each student to make initial contact with each professional. Each student should be able to send the instructor the 10 professionals contacted and why each was contacted. No more than a page of information should be submitted to the instructor.

## Steps To Confidence

35. Building confidence and belief. Some of us are low achievers, and some of us are high achievers. It is as simple as that. As an instructor, creating a learning atmosphere that is great for growth and enhances a student's self-concept is essential. The objective of this exercise is to get students to feel good about themselves. Many teachers who are underpaid or have multiple responsibilities can neglect a student's mental health. Mental health is enhanced with confidence. Confidence comes from a wide range of support, and instructors are a large support system and creators of a game plan for student success. 5 things that build confidence and 5 things that make you as a student want to believe you can be successful? Each student should be able to write down 10 things, not just a one-word answer or a simple sentence, but a well-thought-out page of information. Give each student at least 15 minutes and ensure they are taking their time developing this list.

## Being Versatile

36. Being comfortable in uncomfortable situations. In a class, everyone should circle up together, hold hands, stand on one leg and hold it for 30 seconds. They have 3 chances to achieve it if they do give them something small like Hershey's candy or small bubble gum. The objective of this task is to create a reward system. In life, there is always a reward system. If you work hard at an entry-level position after college, you may have an opportunity to move up in that company. If the class can complete this task together, they deserve a reward.

## Time Management

37. Why should an individual be on time for work? Should a person be fired if they are late? Ask these 2 questions. Require at least 3 participants for each question. The objective is for the class to devise an effective solution to employees' abuse of not following their work schedules. At the end of the discussion, there should be an understanding of why people should be punctual and practice good time management.

## Understanding Credit

38. Financial literacy and credit. Let your students understand the importance of keeping their bank account in good condition and understanding what credit score they should need. This task is simple to start off by asking the class why it is important to have good financial literacy and credit. When you have completed that. Let them know the breakdown of scores: (300-579) poor, (580-669) fair, (670-739) good, (740-799) very good, and (800-850) excellent. The objective is for the instructor to have a brief 15-20 minutes discussion of what a good credit score is and a good understanding of the importance of balancing finances and how it will lead to a successful outcome. The discussion should talk about ways your life can be negatively impacted by poor financial management. For example, not qualifying for a home, car, or loan. There also can be repossession of property in extreme circumstances. This exercise is vital to many young people looking for a bright future. Many of us are not taught this essential skill at a young age, which should be emphasized in classes nationwide.

Outdoor activity. A scavenger hunt or community activity involves interacting with one person outside the normal body of people. The scavenger hunt should be prepared beforehand and should consist of a piece of paper for every student to find, which consists of a different career.

## Career Goals

39. Give each student a particular career they need to find on the paper and make sure they are able to work well with each other for the common goal. The second activity, instead of the hunt, is asking a person in the community or institution what career they are in and how they got there. The objective is to familiarize the students with different careers than the one they are focused on attaining.

## Communication

40. Mental health and communication have been focal points as there has been a need for help worldwide. Many people who have a hard time struggle to communicate their struggles. Ensuring that a learning experience involves a portion of mental development can be essential to enhancing the students' performance. Ask your students to get into 2 groups. Give them 5 minutes to discuss. The exercise should take 20 minutes. The question of discussion is how can a person be more mentally sane? It may sound crazy but see what the students come up with. Ensure you embrace their responses and encourage them to work on their meditation, seek social support and find something that allows them to clear their mind. For example, the gym can help someone's mental health. When people put on their music and are locked into their gym routine, they can develop inner peace. At the end of the discussion, each student should be able to discuss one thing that will keep their mental health at peace.

## Effective Thinking

41. As the semester winds down and there's time for evaluation and finals. Students need to be encouraged with effective thinking. The last few weeks of exercise should be more engaging for future plans. For this exercise, simply ask what now? Further explain that each student should be able to stand up, be confident with public speaking, and explain what their short-term goal is. The objective is to hear an immediate goal, not something over time but something a student can complete when they leave. Feel free as an instructor to reconstruct that question and add more detail to get a more in-depth explanation.

## Academic Success

42. Why is academic success based on deliberate practice? There should be a 10-minute discussion at the end of class.

    Objective: summarize the students' knowledge from previous learning.

## Financial Literacy

43. How does financial literacy impact society? There should be a 10-minute discussion at the end of class.

    Objective: summarize the students' knowledge from previous learning.

## Be Open

44. How is being open to differences allow you to be a great achiever? There should be a 10-minute discussion at the end of class.

    Objective: summarize the students' knowledge from previous learning.

## Career Aspirations

45. How long does it take to get into the career of your dreams? There should be a 10-minute discussion at the end of class.

    Objective: summarize the students' knowledge from previous learning.

## Group Work

46. How does group work play a role in the success of an outcome? There should be a 10-minute discussion at the end of class.

    Objective: summarize the students' knowledge from previous learning.

## 30 Seconds

47. All students should close their eyes for 30 seconds. Think of 5 ways they can change for the better. Write it down and then speak it to existence in front of the class.

## Journal

48. The last exercise is a journal. Provide each student a 30–365-day journal. This choice is up to the instructor. The journal is to provide effective strategies for achieving day-to-day goals. Each student should write what they need to do that day and how they will achieve it. This is a daily journal, so there should be enough space to complete this task. This is a gift that you can give your students to ensure they know you are with them in their future endeavors and that you value their success after completing the course requirement.

# AUTHOR'S BIOGRAPHY

I am an Immigrant Masters student who grew up in Toronto, Canada. Raised in a single-parent home. I lived in Toronto until I was 13. I was having some trouble in school and was on my way to either being in a juvenile detention center or ending up dead. My mom moved me out of the low-income area and provided me (add "with") a better life in a smaller city, where I began to play football and focus my aggression on something productive. Fast forward 5 years, I was in college trying to make a way for my family.

I was an all-league offensive tackle in California and had over 20 division 1 offers and interest approaching my graduation from junior college. I had to go back to my country to work because I could not afford to graduate. The 20 schools turned into 1. North Carolina Agricultural and Technical State University is where I attended on a full scholarship. I was committed to the program for 2 years.

When the COVID-19 pandemic started, the upcoming season was canceled, which was my last year of division 1 eligibility. There was no pro day, no scouts, and I ultimately fell off the radar to play professional football. I continued to work out and kept focused on finishing college. I attended Western Colorado University a year later to graduate with my degree and finish what I started in junior college.

Now I am working on my master's degree at Arizona State University and looking forward to a career in sports psychology with aspirations to eventually work with a professional football team giving them mental health tips and ways to perform at their best on and off the field.

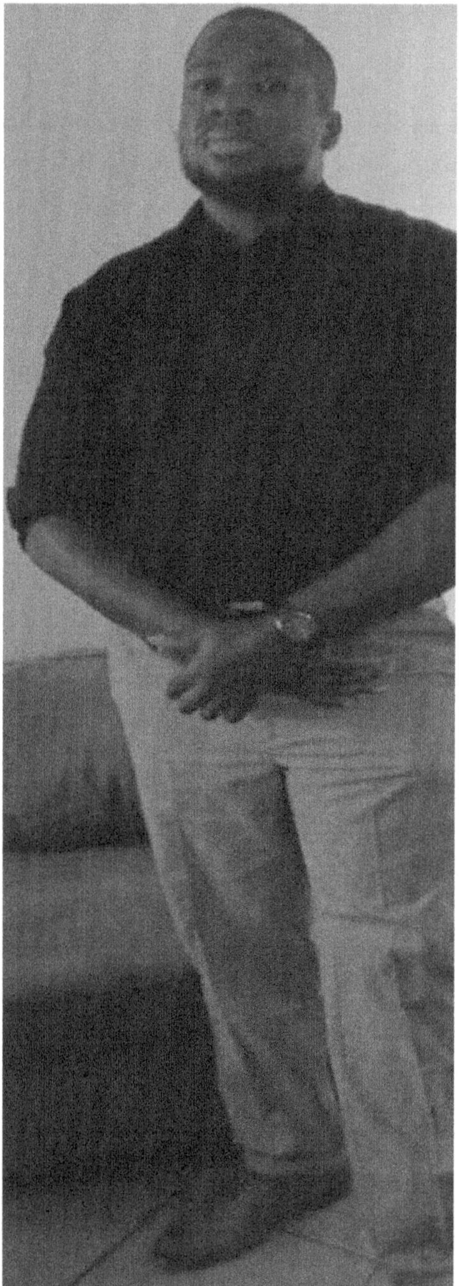

# READERS' NOTEPAD